ASSESSING, PLANNING & MONITORING CARE

FOR NURSING ASSOCIATES

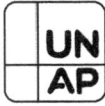

UN | UNDERSTANDING
AP | NURSING ASSOCIATE
PRACTICE

ASSESSING, PLANNING & MONITORING CARE

FOR NURSING ASSOCIATES

Hazel Cowls
Sarah Tobin

LM Learning Matters

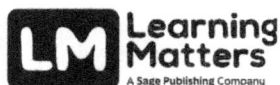

Learning Matters
LM
A Sage Publishing Company

1 Oliver's Yard
55 City Road
London EC1Y 1SP

2455 Teller Road
Thousand Oaks
California 91320

10th Floor, Emaar Capital Tower 2
MG Road, Sikanderpur, Sector 26
Gurugram, Haryana – 122002
India

8 Marina View Suite 43-053
Asia Square Tower 1
Singapore 018960

Library of Congress Control Number: 2025943506

British Library Cataloguing in Publication Data

A catalogue record for this book is available from the British Library

Editor: Martha Cunneen
Senior project editor: Chris Marke
Project management: TNQ Tech Pvt. Ltd.
Marketing manager: Ruslana Khatagova
Cover design: Wendy Scott
Typeset by: TNQ Tech Pvt. Ltd.

ISBN 978-1-5296-9063-7
ISBN 978-1-5296-9062-0 (pbk)

Contents

About the authors   ix
Acknowledgement   xi

Introduction   1

1   Accountability   5

2   Working in partnership with people   23

3   Bio-psycho-social healthcare assessment   39

4   Understanding assessment tools   57

5   How and when to monitor and escalate care   73

6   The principles and theories of planning nursing care   89

7   Consider the wider determinants of health when providing and monitoring care   109

8   The importance of sensitive and compassionate assessment and planning for
    all people   125

References   143
Index   151

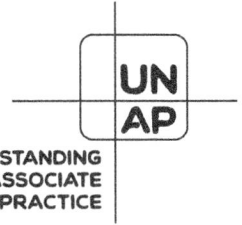

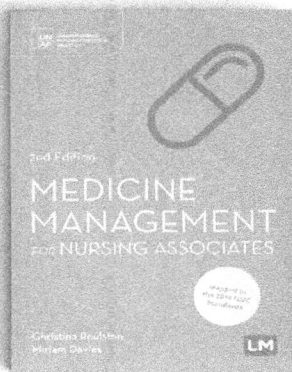

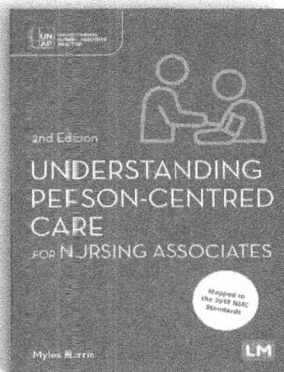

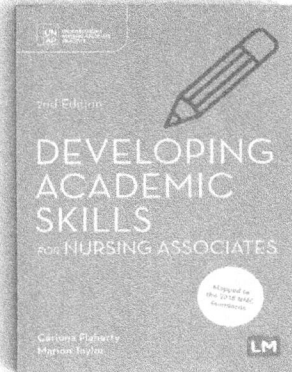

About the authors

Hazel Cowls is a lecturer in adult nursing at the University of Plymouth School of Nursing and Midwifery. Hazel is a Registered Nurse, and she has 28 years' experience in clinical practice, including 2 years' teaching experience in practice. She has 8 years' experience teaching across nursing associate and undergraduate nursing programmes. Hazel has completed MSc in Contemporary Healthcare (Education).

Sarah Tobin is an NMC registered adult nurse, mental health nurse and registered nurse teacher and has worked in emergency care, elderly care, oncology and cancer screening, as well as gastroenterology. Currently working as a Lecturer in Adult Nursing at the University of Plymouth, she also continues to work as a Clinical Nurse Specialist at Torbay and South Devon NHS Foundation Trust. Sarah's MSc and subsequent PhD research focused on defining compassion in healthcare and how this can be demonstrated. The findings confirmed her belief that compassionate care is a clinically relevant and important skill that all healthcare staff need to demonstrate.

Lisa-Marie Rowe is an experienced Lecturer of Adult Nursing and the Programme Lead for Nursing Associates at the University of Plymouth where she achieved her MSc in Advanced Professional Practice. A proud Queen's Nurse, she is passionate about the delivery of gold standard, person-centered care, a philosophy she carries into her teaching and writing. Lisa-Marie began her career as a community nurse in Cornwall, where she continues to live today.

Acknowledgement

Thank you to Lanto Bickerstaff and Sarah Brown who were willing to share their experiences of planning and monitoring patient care while working as registered nursing associates.

Introduction

Who is this book for?

This book has been written to help support and inform student nursing associates (SNAs) as it makes very direct links to the relevant Nursing and Midwifery Council (NMC) Standards of Proficiency (NMC, 2024). However, the content is applicable to nurses in any field and at any level of their continuing educational endeavours. The nursing associate role is a separate profession and has a different set of responsibilities as defined by the NMC. Nursing associates contribute to the ongoing assessment of a person's needs, inform and contribute to care plans and will provide and monitor care.

About the book

Nursing Associates (NAs) are in the unique position of being able to practise across all fields of nursing with a single qualification. It is important therefore to maximise those skills that are universal, transferable and applicable – providing and monitoring care are essential skills. The NA role was established to 'bridge the gap' between the healthcare assistant and the registered nurse and this is very evident in the collegiate way that underpins nursing assessments. Assessment informs care plans and these need to be followed, monitored and updated as required – NAs have a vital role within this process.

Each chapter can stand alone and act as a clear and informative resource to help develop your understanding of why planning and monitoring patient care is important. However, taken as a whole, the eight chapters form a comprehensive exploration of assessing need, providing and monitoring care, the underpinning theory in relation to the wider nursing profession and, specifically, the new and ever-developing role of the NA.

The authors have aimed to make the chapters engaging and informative and to challenge you to think about your nursing practice. NAs are a valuable member of the multi-disciplinary team and may need to work alone, with people in their own home, a community setting or in hospital. Individual care needs may fluctuate over time, and the NA needs to be able to recognise clinical changes, be able to provide and monitor care, and recognise when to escalate care.

Book structure

1. Accountability

In this chapter, you will explore how the NMC Code of Standards of Proficiency (2024) and the Code of Professional Standards (2024) link to your accountability and your role in assessing, planning and monitoring care whether that is a primary activity or under supervision. You will become aware of legal, statutory and ethical frameworks and how these impact on your practice. You will explore the importance of personhood and the need to provide person-centred and holistic care.

2. Working in partnership with people

In this chapter, you will build on the concept of person-centred care and family-centred care. Nursing Associates continually monitor the individual health needs of people within their care working in partnership with people, their family and carers. SNAs and RNAs contribute to ongoing assessment and recognise when to refer to others within the wider multi-disciplinary team (MDT) for input and further assessment. There will be links to the importance of interprofessional and inter-agency working to ensure the provision of effective care that is 'joined-up'.

3. Bio-psycho-social healthcare assessment

In this chapter, you will explore the principles of a bio-psycho-social assessment and why this model supports a person-centred approach. You will see how this has developed to include a spiritual assessment of a person's needs across their lifespan and what is meant by a 'spiritual' model. You will begin to recognise the importance of inter-disciplinary working in order to meet the bio-psycho-social needs of an individual.

4. Understanding assessment tools

In this chapter, we will introduce the SNA and RNA to relevant assessment tools used in clinical practice. Assessment tools can support the initial assessment of a person's health as well as ongoing monitoring. The validity and specificity of different tools used in a variety of clinical settings and across different fields of nursing and a person's lifespan will also be discussed. Examples of assessment tools have been included and contextualised in case studies.

5. How and when to monitor and escalate care

In this chapter, you will be building on work from earlier chapters by looking at the underpinning theory of clinical reasoning and clinical decision-making. You will review assessment tools and 'track and trigger' systems that can support your clinical decision-making. As a SNA or RNA, you will work closely with individuals, their family or carers as well as the wider multi-disciplinary team. Therefore, you will consider effective ways of communicating and working with others. Through case studies, you will explore how you can contribute to ongoing assessments and escalation of care.

6. The principles and theories of planning nursing care

In this chapter, you will continue to build on your knowledge of the principles and theories of planning nursing care. The SNA and RNA will make an important contribution to the safe and effective planning of nursing care. Whilst the accountability for care provision may well rest with the RN, it is imperative not to underestimate the role of the SNA/RNA in the planning process. This chapter will therefore cover the nursing process (Assessment, Systematic Diagnosis, Implementation, Recheck and Evaluations) as well as introduce you to three nursing models. You will be introduced to care pathways and care bundles and explore how evidence supports clinical practice.

7. Consider the wider determinants of health when assessing and monitoring care

In this chapter, you will explore the concept of the wider determinants of health, the social determinants of health and health disparities in more detail. You will review relevant publications such as The Marmot Review; 10 years on the Marmot Review and be introduced to models such as Dahlgren and Whitehead (1993). Developing an understanding of these wider determinants of health will enable SNAs and RNAs to consider the challenges people face. Understanding care needs in a wider context ensures planned care is relevant and realistic. You will look at initiatives that aim to improve health in individuals and communities. The case studies provided will help to put the theory into context.

8. The importance of sensitive and compassionate assessment and planning for all people

In this chapter, you will develop an understanding of compassion and how this underpins safe and effective care provision. You will explore how needs assessment and the planning of care that is based on compassionate principles can be delivered. You will learn the importance of compassionate cultures and how you can contribute to them and in turn provide compassionate care. The importance of compassionate input when caring for those at the end of life and the concept of advanced care planning will be considered.

Requirements for the NMC standards of proficiency for nursing associates

The Nursing and Midwifery Council (NMC) has established standards of proficiency to be met by applicants to different parts of the register, and these are the standards it considers necessary for safe and effective practice. This book is structured so that it will help you to understand and meet the proficiencies required for entry to the NMC register as a nursing associate. The relevant proficiencies are presented at the start of each chapter so that you can clearly see which ones the chapter addresses. The proficiencies have been designed to be generic, so they apply to all fields of nursing and all care settings. This is because all nursing associates must be able to meet the needs of any person they encounter in their practice regardless of their stage of life or health challenges, whether these are mental, physical, cognitive or behavioural.

This book includes the latest standards for 2024 onwards, taken from the *Standards of Proficiency for nursing associates* (NMC, 2024).

Learning features

Textbooks can be intimidating, and learning from reading text is not always easy. However, this series has been designed specifically to help the nursing associate learn from the books within it. By using a variety of learning features throughout the book, they will help you to develop your understanding and ability to apply theory to practice, whilst remaining engaging and breaking the text up into manageable chunks. This book contains activities, case studies, theory summary boxes, further reading, useful websites and other materials to enable you to participate in your own learning. The book cannot provide all the answers – but instead provides a good outline of the most important information and helps you build a framework for your own learning.

Final word

We hope that you find the information in this book supports your academic studies and enables you to develop your skills as an RNA. Remember to draw on the knowledge and experience of others that you work alongside as it is an essential for all registered nurses, registered nursing associates and midwives to support colleagues and to help them to develop their professional competence and confidence.

Accountability

Sarah Tobin

NMC *STANDARDS FOR PROFICIENCY FOR NURSING ASSOCIATES*

This Chapter will address the following platforms and proficiencies.

Platform 1: Being an accountable practitioner

1.1   understand and act in accordance with The Code: Professional standards of practice and behaviour for nurses, midwives and nursing associates, and fulfil all registration requirements.

1.2   understand and apply relevant legal, regulatory and governance requirements, policies, and ethical frameworks, including any mandatory reporting duties, to all areas of practice.

1.7   describe the principles of research and how research findings are used to inform evidence-based practice.

1.17   safely demonstrate evidence-based practice in all skills and procedures stated in Annexes A and B.

Platform 3: Provide and monitor care

3.1   demonstrate an understanding of human development from conception to death, to enable delivery of person-centred safe and effective care.

Chapter aims

After reading this chapter you will be able to:

- Understand how the NMC Code of Standards of Proficiency (2024) and the Code of Professional Standards (2024) link to your accountability and your role as a nursing associate in assessment and planning.
- Better understand the concept of best interests and of personhood and how this links to the provision of holistic care.
- Make the link between professional practice and evidence-based thinking and how this relates to accountability.
- Be aware of the importance of legal, statutory, governance and ethical frameworks and how this impacts assessment, planning and monitoring of care.

Introduction

This book highlights the importance and impact of assessment, planning, and monitoring in the provision of effective and person-centred care. Nurses are responsible for these functions for the patients within their care and are therefore accountable for how this is achieved. Accountability means that you are answerable for your decisions and practice and the organisation that dictates the standards that underpin that practice is The Nursing and Midwifery Council (NMC). In fact, the NMC Standards of Proficiency for Nursing Associates (2024) states that whilst *'Nursing Associates are a new profession'* they are, as with all registered professionals, *'accountable for their practice'*. Indeed, the entirety of the first platform of these Standards relates to the requirement to be an accountable professional, describing 17 elements that must be met by the point of registration to demonstrate this accountability. As with Registered Nurses and Midwives, a Student Nursing Associate (SNA) or a Registered Nursing Associate (RNA) also needs to comply with the NMC Code of Professional Standards and Behaviours (The Code) 2018. The Code (2018) also highlights the importance of accountability, stating that, *'all of the professions we regulate exercise professional judgement and are accountable for their work'*. The concept of accountability will be explored more fully within this chapter and also in elements throughout this book as it impacts and underpins all aspects of practice.

Accountability, responsibility, and delegation and how this links to assessment and planning

Perhaps the most important idea linked to the concept of accountability is that of safety – the key requirement to 'do no harm'. It is sobering and very important to remember that the first line of The Code (2018) states that the NMC *'exists to protect the public'*. . ..full stop! This mission statement is explained by linking the requirements within the Code (2018) and the relevant Standards for Proficiency to the fitness of individuals to be called Nursing Associates or Registered Nurses. You need to understand, adhere to, and demonstrate competence with these regulations and standards to legally merit the title Nursing Associate.

There is an important consideration for RNAs however as, whilst they are registered, professional nurses, they are not Registered Nurses (RNs) and this can lead to some confusion about their role and where accountability lies. The NMC has devised a helpful graphic which demonstrates the key differences in terms of role between an RNA and an RN (see Figure 1.1) and, from looking at this, you may believe that RNAs do not have a role in assessing and planning care for patients. You would be wrong. Language matters and, whilst the RN may take a **lead** in these roles, all members of the nursing team and specifically RNAs will carry out assessments, *'provide and monitor care'* and therefore have significant impact on any plan of care. Every time you measure a patient's observations, assess their pressure areas, take a blood sample or record how much they have eaten or drunk you are assessing their needs. Accurate reporting and record keeping of assessment findings will then underpin planned care and, importantly, any changes that may be required to that plan. Nursing is a dynamic and skilled job; the interaction between nurse and patient is vitally important and your ability to respond and adapt to patient needs is integral to ensuring that they receive the correct care.

Nursing associate 6 platforms	Registered nurse 7 platforms
Be an accountable professional	Be an accountable professional
Promoting health and preventing ill health	Promoting health and preventing ill health
Provide and monitor care	Provide and evaluate care
Working in teams	Leading and managing nursing care and working in teams
Improving safety and quality of care	Improving safety and quality of care
Contributing to integrated care	Coordinating care
	Assessing needs and planning care

Figure 1.1   The key differences between and RN and a RNA

Delegation is a key concept that influences your role in assessing and planning and shows how accountability can be a shared responsibility. While an RN may be accountable for the care provided to a group of patients, they will need to delegate aspects of patient care to appropriate colleagues. If an RN delegates the role of assessment, the completion or updating of a care plan or subsequent monitoring to the RNA, as it is agreed to be within their scope of practice, then the RNA, by accepting these duties, takes on the accountability as well.

Activity 1.1   Research

Use the internet to access the NMC document, Delegation and Accountability: Supplementary Information to the NMC Code. The link is here:
www.nmc.org.uk/globalassets/sitedocuments/nmc-publications/delegation-and-accountability-supplementary-information-to-the-nmc-code.pdf
Read this short, six-page document and list the four requirements in relation to accepting delegated activities. Then consider the implications of these, described in the next section of the document. Did you realise that both the person who delegates aspects of care but also the person who accepts that delegation share the accountability?

Some key concepts and answers are included at the end of this chapter.

If accountability means to be answerable, then who do we answer to?

Anyone who is registered with a professional body such as the NMC agrees to abide by the standards and proficiencies that merit that registration. An RNA is therefore accountable to uphold the NMC Standards of Proficiency (2024) and The Code of professional standards (2018) and would be required to answer to the NMC for any breaches.

Those who provide healthcare, whether the over-arching organisation or the individual employed by them, are also accountable to both the criminal and civil law of the country. So, healthcare staff, whether qualified or not, need to ensure that their actions conform to legal requirements. This concept also relates to things you may not do, omissions, as not doing something for someone when it is needed can also result in harm. The law describes this as a 'duty of care' and all nurses owe this duty to their patients and at a higher level than that expected of a member of the public who does not have their knowledge, training and expertise.

The vast majority of nurses will not work independent of an employing organisation, whether NHS or a private provider such as a nursing home, GP Practice or hospice. This means that you are also accountable to your employer and must abide by your contract of employment which will state the terms and conditions of your practice.

Finally, and perhaps most importantly, you are accountable to the patients that entrust themselves and their care to your keeping. We look after the most vulnerable people in our communities, the frail, the dying, the confused and the frightened. Healthcare staff possess expert knowledge which patients may find difficult to understand, and we use drugs and equipment that can help and heal but which, when used incorrectly, can harm and even kill. This means that we must exercise the highest levels of responsibility to be knowledgeable and competent. This then underpins our ability to account for our decisions, actions, and omissions.

A quick mention about the idea of vicarious liability – this means that employers hold the legal liability for any acts or omissions of their employees that cause harm to a patient if carried out as part of their employment. Consequently if you make a mistake at work and a patient were to complain or even sue for damages then your employer would be liable to address this. That does not mean you do not remain accountable and if the mistake was because of some fault on your part, you could still be required to answer to the employer, to a court of law, or to your regulatory body.

Case study 1.1: Penny

Penny is an RNA working in a GP Practice where she enjoys a significant level of autonomy within her daily practice. This has resulted from support to attend a number of different advanced training days to equip her to undertake additional clinical roles which have been reflected within her contract of employment. One such role is to carry out cervical screening (smear tests) for women who are invited to take part in the GP-led national screening programme.

During one screening clinic she meets Stephanie, a 36-year-old lady who is coming to have the procedure for the first time. Stephanie is clearly anxious and seems very distracted, she asks Penny lots of questions about the procedure which Penny answers with care and knowledge. Stephanie then asks whether Penny thinks that she ought to have a coil fitted as she is concerned about taking the contraceptive pill again, she and her husband have completed their family and do not want any further children. Whilst Penny has no specific family planning training, she discusses options and ideas whilst carrying out and completing the smear. Penny feels that, on balance, a coil would be the best option for Stephanie. At the end of the appointment Stephanie feels a lot happier and seems visibly more relaxed, she states that Penny's advice has been really helpful, and she will go ahead and book in with the practice RN in order to get a coil fitted. Penny offers to make the appointment for her before she leaves.

Activity 1.2   Critical thinking

1. Were there any clues that Stephanie's appointment may have been more than a routine meeting?
2. Was it appropriate for Penny to offer advice to Stephanie?
3. What, if any, are the possible implications of Stephanie attending the appointment with the RN for the coil fitting?
4. If you believe Penny should have taken an alternative approach to the appointment, what could she have done differently?

A model answer is provided at the end of the chapter.

There is therefore a very real link between competence and accountability. This will be explored more in the final section of this chapter, but you need to consider a very important concept; namely, the requirement to act within and to the level of your competence.

The concept of 'best interests'

Platform 1 of the Standards of Proficiency for Nursing Associates (2024) begins with the statement that Nursing Associates demonstrate accountability by acting *'in the best interests of people, putting them first and providing nursing care that is person-centred, safe, and compassionate'.* So, what are the 'best interests' of people? Generally speaking, when a person is able to decide for themselves, best interests are the decisions that they make about their own healthcare needs. This requires them to be appropriately informed and supported in order to make such decisions.

An important legal guideline that you need to be aware of is known as The Mental Capacity Act (MCA), 2005. This is government legislation which exists to support and protect people aged over 16 in England and Wales who may not be in a position to make their own decisions. An Act of Parliament which has been passed by both houses of Parliament and given the consent of the monarch, such as the MCA, creates or modifies a law. So, the guidelines in the MCA are not negotiable – they are legally binding on healthcare providers. The Act states that in order to be able to make their own decisions a person needs to be able to:

- Understand information provided to them;
- Retain the information long enough to make a decision;
- Weigh up the positives and negatives of the information;
- Communicate their decision – in any way that can be understood.

If any or all of these elements are compromised, then the person may lack the capacity to make their own decisions and relevant healthcare professionals may need to make decisions on the person's behalf and in their best interests.

Understand the theory - MCA: Best interest principles

Section 4 of the Mental Capacity Act has a best interests checklist. This outlines what someone needs to consider before taking an action or making a decision for anyone who has been identified as lacking capacity. They must consider all the relevant circumstances and, in particular, take the following steps to decide what is in a person's best interest.

1. Consider whether it is likely that the person will at some time have capacity in relation to the matter in question, and if so, when that is likely to be.
2. Must, so far as is reasonably practicable, permit and encourage the person to participate or to improve their ability to participate, as fully as possible in any act done for them and any decision affecting them.
3. If the decision relates to life-sustaining treatment they must not, in considering whether treatment is in the best interests of the person concerned, be motivated by a desire to bring about their death.
4. Must consider, so far as is reasonably possible, the person's past and present wishes and feelings (and in particular, any relevant written statement made by them when they had capacity), any beliefs and values that would be likely to influence their decision if they had capacity, and any other factors that they would be likely to consider if able to do so.
5. Must take into account, if it is practicable and appropriate to consult them, the views of:

   - anyone named by the person as someone to be consulted on the matter in question;
   - anyone engaged in caring for that person or interested in their welfare;
   - anyone with a lasting power of attorney granted by the person;
   - any deputy appointed for the person by the court.

It might be useful to consider what actually is a 'person'... if we are going to contribute to making decisions about what is best for a person, let's think about what defines a 'person'.

Activity 1.3 Reflection

Before you read the next section on the 'theory' of personhood take a minute or two to consider what you think makes a person? You will have your own ideas and thoughts, perhaps you follow a specific religion, and this influences your beliefs about personhood. You may have had personal or work experiences or conversations that impacted or even altered your opinion. Perhaps you have never really given the idea much thought at all – whatever the situation is, now is the time to gather your thoughts and consider your understanding of 'what is a person'?

As this is a reflective activity, no model answer has been provided. Please now read some of the theoretical ideas that follow – do these confirm or change your ideas?

The concept of personhood

The question, 'what is a person?' may seem fairly straightforward at first glance but it is a conundrum which has challenged some of the greatest thinkers across the centuries. And why should it matter? Well, much is written about person-centred care but without stopping to consider the nature of personhood it is challenging to understand what person-centred care might be. Also, healthcare itself can be a controversial concept, dealing with and impacted by arguments related to euthanasia, abortion, gender identity and the use of animals in experiments. All of these ideas link to the basic understanding of what constitutes being a person.

First, there is a distinction between being 'human', a biological concept linked to DNA and being a 'person', a moral or philosophical concept linked to characteristics. And these defining characteristics have, over history, meant that those from different ethnic backgrounds, those who were enslaved, those with disabilities, and even those who were women, have been denied the same level of personhood as others. If a society controls the definition of personhood, then they can include or exclude those who do not meet these characteristics.

The philosopher, Mary Anne Warren (1946–2010) suggested that the following criteria could be used to define a person:

- Consciousness (of objects and events external and/or internal to the being), and in particular the capacity to feel pain;
- Reasoning (the capacity to solve new and relatively complex problems);
- Self-motivated activity (activity which is relatively independent of either genetic or direct external control);
- The capacity to communicate, by whatever means, messages of an indefinite variety of types, that is, not just with an indefinite number of possible contents, but on indefinitely many possible topics;
- The presence of self-concepts and self-awareness, either individual or racial, or both. (Warren, 1973).

Activity 1.4 Critical thinking

Using the criteria set out by Mary Anne Warren think about the following examples:

1. A foetus that has reached eight months' gestation.
2. An adult who, following an accident, is in a persistent vegetative state.
3. A chimpanzee.
4. Someone with advanced dementia.
5. A person in a coma on life-support in Intensive Care.

Which of these scenarios, when judged by these criteria would qualify as a 'person'? Is there a difference between being a person and being human? What does it matter anyway?

A model answer is provided at the end of the chapter.

Some interesting legal cases that help determine the impact of personhood in healthcare

In the whole of the UK, with some minor differences across the regions, some laws are established when judges have to rule in cases that do not seem to 'fit' with established legal precedents. These cases and the rulings made then serve to act as guides in future, similar cases.

A significant case was that of Tony Bland who in 1989 at 17 years of age went to watch a football match held at the Hillsborough stadium. A fatal crush occurred when fans became trapped resulting in 766 people injured and 97 fatalities, one of which was Tony, who died almost four years later. Tony was crushed resulting in catastrophic injuries which left him with irreversible damage to his brain leaving him in a persistent vegetative state. The opinion of all those caring for him, and that of his parents, was that his body was being kept alive by artificial nutrition, hydration, and excellent care and that there was no chance that he would emerge from his vegetative state. At the time his doctors were told that as the law stood, they would be liable to a charge of murder if they withdrew treatment and Tony died. The case was therefore heard in court, known as Airedale National Health Service Trust v Bland [1993] AC 789. The judges ruled that it was unlawful to intentionally cause death but that it was legal for treatment that was not in Tony's best interests to be withdrawn. As the treatment being given to Tony had no prospect of improving his condition it could be deemed futile and as there was no interest for Tony in continuing it, it was lawful to stop. Whilst this case remains controversial to some, it is the legal basis that supports withholding or withdrawing treatment assessed as not being in a person's best interests.

The case of a patient who was detained in a secure hospital (Re C, Adult, refusal of treatment, [1994] ER 819) determined that a person who had a significant mental illness could still make a decision about their healthcare. 'C' had paranoid schizophrenia which, amongst other delusions, led him to believe he had a successful international career in medicine. Following an injury, he developed gangrene in a foot wound which led a vascular surgeon to conclude that without amputation 'C' had only a 15 per cent chance of survival. 'C' declined the surgery believing the doctors to be wrong and even if they weren't he 'rather die with two feet than live with one'. A judge ruled that 'C' met the criteria to make a decision – he could understand and retain treatment information, believe it and weigh it in a balanced way to make a choice. So, 'C' kept his foot and was treated conservatively, going on to live for another 10 years before dying of an unrelated problem.

Finally, just because a decision seems to be unwise, a person still has the right to make it if they have capacity. In the case of 'B' (Re B, Adult, refusal of treatment, [2002] ER 449). Ms B, a women aged 43, suffered a sudden and catastrophic illness which resulted in paralysis from the neck down leaving her reliant on a ventilator, she could speak using a speech valve – there was no prospect of recovery. Ms B repeatedly requested that the ventilator be removed as she felt her life was not one she could or would ever accept. There was understandable disquiet at the prospect of switching off the equipment that was keeping her alive, so judicial review was sought. The judges ruled that as long as a person has capacity then their wishes need to be respected irrespective of the outcome and the clinicians' views as to the best interests of the patient are, in this circumstance, irrelevant. Therefore, the ventilator was removed, and Ms B subsequently died.

These are just three cases that serve to explain some of the complexity relating to how a person can be viewed and how it is possible to establish best interests. There are many more that could be described that have equal impact. If you are interested why not do some further research into case law and how it impacts health care. Links to some additional resources can be found at the end of the chapter.

Back to personhood quickly...

So, perhaps the way to address the idea of 'what is a person'? is to consider that whoever you care for is a unique individual, no matter what their capabilities, no matter what their beliefs, no matter how they think or feel. If we agree with this sentiment than we must equally hold with the notion that care must be tailored to the needs of each individual as there can be no guideline or pathway (however evidence-based) that will work for 100 per cent or people 100 per cent of the time. So, in order to ensure that people receive the care that they need we need to make certain that they are adequately assessed.

Activity 1.5   Reflection

You are a SNA working in a busy Emergency Department; the team are informed that there has been a significant road traffic accident and number of badly injured patients are being brought in. You and your colleagues are asked to care for one patient who was thrown from a motorbike during the incident; James is a 19-year-old young man who initially looks as if he has suffered only minor injuries. However, his condition rapidly deteriorates, and it is determined that he has likely ruptured his spleen and is bleeding internally – he needs urgent surgery to save his life. The surgeon comes to assess him and to gain consent, the consent includes the necessity to provide both intra-operative and possibly post-operative blood transfusions. James states that he is a practising Jehovah's Witness and refuses consent to receive any blood products, the surgeon is clear that he believes James may not survive without the transfusions. Despite being very unwell James appears to be clear in his understanding of the consequences of his decision and is adamant in his refusal.

You are asked to stay with James and monitor his observations as he waits to go to theatre. You talk to James and reassure him as much as possible, he is clearly very frightened although does not appear to doubt his decision.

How would you feel in this situation? What are your personal views about a patient's right to refuse treatment even if this might result in harm or even death?

As these are very personal questions which will result in unique and personal responses (you also have your own 'personhood' after all) no model answer is provided. However, some resources and guidelines will be suggested in the answer section at the end of the chapter.

Person-centred and holistic care - the link to assessment

The Standards (2024) state that RNAs must *'provide person-centred, safe and compassionate care'*. We have established that the concept of 'person' is far from straightforward but what about person-centred care? What does this oft-stated description of care provision actually mean? Another book in this series, *Understanding Person-Centred Care for Nursing Associates* by Myles Harris (2024, 2nd edition) provides a comprehensive analysis of this concept and is to be recommended. I will therefore confine myself to a definition and a discussion about the link to assessment.

Definition would seem simple, but as with personhood, is complicated by many different theories and ideas. The NHS (2024) suggests that being person-centred is *'about focussing care on the needs of individuals. Ensuring that people's preferences, needs and values guide clinical decisions, and providing care that is respectful of and responsive to them.'* Some feel this encompasses the broader idea of patient engagement and ensuring patients are involved at all levels of decision-making, not just for their health but also in health policy.

The Health Foundation (2016) highlights the importance of this in the light of the significant increase in older people and of people who are living with and having to manage chronic, long-term health conditions.

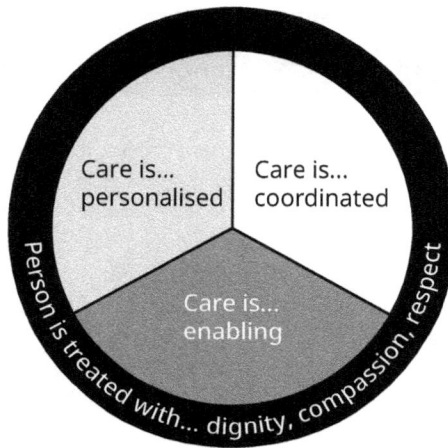

Figure 1.2   The four principles of person-centred care

Source: The Health Foundation (2016).

According to the Health Foundation (2016), instead of trying to define the idea it is better to describe the underlying principles. These are demonstrated in Figure 1.2 – *'Whatever the specific care or interventions a person receives, it should be done with these principles in mind. Any example of person-centred care, within any health care experience, will involve a combination of these principles'*. The NMC Code (2018) emphasises the idea of patient focus and the link to assessment very clearly in all four of the over-arching platforms that frame the standards of conduct. The Standards of Proficiency for Nursing Associates (2024) are equally definitive and the concepts of assessment (however defined), monitoring and the provision of person-centred care are frequently described.

Case study 1.2 Eshan

Eshan is a 62-year-old schoolteacher, he has been admitted to the surgical ward where Lara, a SNA, is currently on placement. The admission is a planned one as Eshan is due to have a hemi-colectomy the next day following a recent diagnosis of colorectal cancer. Lara has been asked to start the admission paperwork for Eshan and to settle him on to the ward. She anticipates that Eshan may be anxious but he appears to be very agitated and it is difficult to ascertain why – Eshan asks if there is a male nurse that he could talk to. Lara immediately goes to find her colleague Mark who is an RNA and also on the shift – he agrees to attend to Eshan.

Later, Lara catches up with Mark and asks him why Eshan was so distressed and why he requested to talk with a male nurse. Mark explains that Eshan is a Sikh (Lara had noticed that he wore a turban) and that his experience so far when he had undergone investigations and had previous treatments had been very challenging for him. He had experienced issues with a recent MRI scan, which almost had to be cancelled and he had read the preoperative patient information leaflet and was very concerned about how his religious needs would be accommodated based on the information that had been given.

Activity 1.6   Research

Read the following resources: www.nes.scot.nhs.uk/media/ay4je0io/multi-faith-resource-for-healthcare-staff.pdf and www.queenscourt.org.uk/resources-training/resource-library/religious-needs-resource/ and then answer the questions below.

- Why do you think Eshan was concerned?
- What aspects of his religious needs were troubling him?
- What do you think Lara could have done as part of his admission assessments to help alleviate some of his concerns?

A model answer is included at the end of this chapter.

The word 'assessment' stems from the Latin word '*assidere*' which means to 'sit beside', so the original concept of assessment was to sit beside someone – what better way to ensure that care is subsequently tailored to their specific needs? When we consider patients as fellow people, members of our community just like 'us', then it is easier to break down barriers and to guard against depersonalisation or the provision of one-size-fits-all care. There is no 'us' and 'them' – just all of 'us'.

Act professionally and the importance of evidence-based thinking

The Standards (2024) state that RNAs need to '*act professionally at all times and use their knowledge and experience to make evidence-based decisions and solve problems*'. As with a number of concepts discussed in this chapter, the concept of professionalism is also difficult to define conclusively. Much is written about what demonstrates professionalism and what it might mean, but perhaps it is sensible to consider what our regulatory body has to say about it.

The NMC Code (2018) is actually, '*The Code: Professional standards of practice and behaviour for nurses, midwives and nursing associates*'. So, as long as our practice adheres to the description of expected behaviour and skills listed within the Code, we can be pretty sure that we are acting professionally. Of course, it is not that simple but, it is a good place to start.

Section 3 of the platform 'Prioritise People' is entitled '*make sure that people's physical, social, and psychological needs are assessed and responded to*'. This requirement can also be described as taking a biopsychosocial approach to healthcare – by viewing a person as having more than simply physical or psychological problems but as comprised of interrelated systems that all need to be assessed for their impact if truly person-centred care is to be provided. This links to the World Health Organization's (1946) original definition of health as '*a state of complete physical, mental and social well-being and not merely the absence of disease*' which remains the definition used to this day (WHO, 2024). This will be discussed more fully in Chapter 3 of this book. It is, however, clear that there is a definite link between assessing a person's needs, of viewing that person as more than the individual sum of their parts, and the NMC expectation of professional practice.

As described above, the NMC also makes it explicit that professional practice is evidence-based, so it is key to also understand how evidence supports the importance of assessment and planning care. The National Institute for Health and Care Excellence (2021) states that assessment is a form of dialogue between client and healthcare practitioner and describes the importance of this dialogue in ensuring patient care is focussed on their individual needs.

A study in 2012 by Rothman et al. demonstrated a strong link between effective assessment and a reduction in both in-hospital and post-discharge mortality. The researchers stated that nursing assessments are both 'clinically meaningful' and 'sensitive indicators of a patient's clinical condition'. Williams (2022) highlights the impact of the introduction of the National Early Warning Score in 2012 citing evidence that demonstrates a reduction of 20 per cent in mortality as a result of sepsis, 50 per cent reductions in cardiac arrests in hospitals and a reduction in the length of hospital stays. And Glasper (2020) describes how Care Quality Commission (CQC) auditors always look for evidence that care provision is tailored to the needs of the individual and that 'at the heart of this requirement is the care plan, and fundamental to this is the robustness of the nursing assessment'. Make no mistake – the RNA role in patient assessment, planning and monitoring is integral to patient safety and to the quality and individualisation of care delivery.

Understand and apply relevant legal, regulatory and governance requirements, policies and ethical frameworks

This is taken from Platform 1, Section 1.2 of the Standards for proficiency (2024) so is not an optional component of your practice, but how does this link to assessing, planning and monitoring care? Well, obviously being aware of how these standards relate to those requirements is a start and has and will be covered in this and subsequent chapters. The Code (NMC, 2018) is also explicit in the link to these activities and the four specific platforms.

Activity 1.7   Know the theory/ research

Access both the Standards of Proficiency (NMC, 2024) and The Code (NMC, 2018) and look through each – highlight each time a link, either directly or indirectly, directs you to the importance or requirement to carry out or contribute to assessing, planning, or monitoring care.

Some examples are included at the end of the chapter.

The purpose of regulation, policy, and standards is ultimately the efficient and safe care of patients – such frameworks exist to promote best practice. Clinical governance is the term used to describe the provision of nationally agreed standards and policies. Scally and Donaldson (1998, p. 61) define clinical governance as *'a system through which NHS organisations are accountable for continuously improving the quality of their services and safeguarding high standards of care by creating an environment in which excellence in clinical care will flourish'*. According to the Royal College of Nursing (RCN, 2024), there are five themes that underpin clinical governance, two of which are 'patient focus' (how services are based on patient need) and 'staff focus' (how staff are developed). Nurses are educated to fulfil the standards laid out by the NMC and the NMC lay out the standards to promote person-centred, effective care provision. Since 2009, the independent organisation the CQC has been responsible for monitoring standards of care in health and social care in England and, as detailed above, makes it clear that person-centredness links very definitely to how patient needs are assessed and subsequently form the basis of any care plan.

Ethical frameworks, however, are concerned with what course of action provides the most appropriate moral outcome, promotes universally accepted 'rules' that underpin conduct and determines how a person, group or organisation understands what is right or wrong. Obviously, the NMC Code (2018) and Standards (2024) provide a framework that supports ethical decision-making but this may not always be comprehensive or specific enough to relate to every situation that a nurse might encounter. As with case law setting precedents to inform the legal status of subsequent patient situations, ethical frameworks can help aid decision-making and support cultural norms when providing care for patients. After all, nurses care, from birth until death, for all of the complex and unique individuals that make up a society and that will inevitably bring challenge and unpredictability.

American philosophers, Beauchamp and Childress, responded to some troubling scientific experiments to try and define a 'common morality' in their first book on biomedical ethics (1979). Taking some centuries-old concepts, they refined them into four principles of biomedical ethics that still form a widely accepted code to help with any consideration about complex or controversial care provision – their original book is now in its eighth iteration last updated in 2019. These principles are universally accepted and can be seen in many ethical codes and standards for medicine, nursing, and allied health professionals.

Understanding the theory

The Four Principles of Biomedical Ethics are:

- **Autonomy** – The right for an individual to make his or her own choice.
- **Beneficence** – The principle of acting with the best interest of the other in mind.
- **Non-maleficence** – The obligation to avoid or minimise inflicting harm on another person. The principle that "above all, do no harm" as stated in most healthcare professional codes of conduct.
- **Justice** – A concept that emphasises fairness and equality among individuals.

As can be seen within these four principles, it would be nigh on impossible to provide people with autonomous choices that underpin their best interests and cause the least amount of harm or restriction if their needs are not assessed and incorporated into an individualised plan of care. All patients need to be cared for in this way, not only the eloquent and educated, so nurses, all nurses, need to understand these principles and advocate for and promote them within their practice.

How your accountable practice links to assessing, planning, and monitoring care

The idea that SNAs and RNAs need to act within their level of competence has been alluded to earlier in the chapter, as has the differences in the roles and responsibilities of an RNA and an RN. This may lead you to believe that it is not within your remit as an SNA/RNA – and therefore your accountability – to assess a patient and, based on this, plan their care. Hopefully, the content of this chapter has changed your mind – SNAs and RNAs are integral to the assessment process and to the planning and subsequent monitoring of care. The Standards (2024) highlight the specific elements of this role, especially within Annex B. However, they also state that *'nursing associates can undertake further education and training and demonstrate additional knowledge and skills, enhancing their competence as other registered professionals routinely do. The roles played by nursing associates will vary from setting to setting, depending on local clinical frameworks, and it may also be shaped by national guidance'*. If the relevant assessment and planning knowledge and skills form part of the expectation and contract of your role or are part of the role delegated to you by a senior colleague, then you will undertake it and be accountable for that practice. At the very least you will need to monitor the care provided to patients and feed this back to the wider team caring for them so that the plan of care can be adhered to or altered as necessary. Nursing care is a dynamic process and requires constant monitoring and adjustment, this is integral to patient assessment and underpins a holistic and adaptive plan of care. Care plans, if they are to provide a responsive schedule of care, must be constantly reviewed and adapted in response to regular and considered monitoring.

Chapter summary

This chapter has outlined some complex but important concepts, the meaning and impact of accountability in your practice has been a main theme throughout. This concept has then been linked to your role in assessing, planning and monitoring care either as a primary activity or one carried out under delegation. The idea of holistic, person-centred care has been explored – by defining personhood and the idea of best interests but also by linking this to assessment and monitoring. The need to fulfil professional obligations both in evidence-based actions but also by adhering to ethical codes has been described. Finally, the link between statutory, governance, and regulatory guidelines and assessment and planning has been made.

Activities: Brief outline answers

Activity 1.1 Research (page 7)

The four responsibilities in relation to accepting delegated activities are:

- Make sure that patient and public safety is not affected. You work within the limits of your competence, exercising your professional 'duty of candour' and raising concerns immediately whenever you come across situations that put patients or public safety at risk.

- Make a timely referral to another practitioner when any action, care, or treatment is required.
- Ask for help from a suitably qualified and experienced health and care professional to carry out any action or procedure that is beyond the limits of your competence.
- Complete the necessary training before carrying out a new role.

The implications of this mean that you must ensure that you understand and can safely carry out any task delegated to you and that it is within your level of competence. You ensure that you have clearly understood what is expected of you including any decisions that may be yours to make and when you may need to update colleagues or escalate care to others.

Activity 1.2 Critical thinking (page 9)

Q1. There were clues that the appointment may not be routine – Stephanie was 36 and was attending for her first cervical smear, the screening programme starts from age 25. Stephanie is 'clearly anxious' and begins the appointment with lots of questions.

Q2. Penny had received additional training to enable her to carry out cervical screening, but she had not received further training in family planning. The advice given was beyond the scope of her competence and it would not therefore have been appropriate.

Q3. The appointment had been made by Penny for Stephanie to have the contraceptive coil fitted, however, this appointment may be wasted if the appropriate information and preparation had not been provided. This was outside of the scope of Penny's competence so these requirements may not have been fulfilled – the implications being a waste of resource and distress and inconvenience to the patient.

Q4. Answering Stephanie's questions about her screening appointment and offering appropriate reassurance and then referring Stephanie to the appropriate colleague for specialist assessment and advice in relation to family planning.

Activity 1.4 Critical thinking (page 11)

When using the criteria set out by Warren, numbers 1, 2, 4, and 5 of the examples provided would not meet the criteria to justify the term 'person'. Example 2, a chimpanzee, would meet the criteria. . ..so there clearly is a difference between being 'human' and being a 'person'. It matters because legislation about very controversial aspects of healthcare such as abortion, euthanasia, autonomy, and resource allocation amongst others, requires definition and clarity. If a human being is not classed as a 'person' then what rights do they have and what responsibility do we? This is why ethical frameworks such as the four principles described by Beauchamp and Childress (2019) can help.

Activity 1.5 Reflection (page 13)

When someone appears to make an 'unwise' choice then the provisions of the Mental Capacity Act (2005) are very helpful – this statutory guideline states that an unwise decision does not imply lack of capacity and if a person is aware of the implications of their decision, then it is their autonomous right to carry out a course of action.

In practice, nursing someone who has made a decision that challenges your understanding and/or beliefs can be distressing. You need to be aware of your own needs and seek help and support as appropriate – a requirement of professional practice.

Activity 1.6 Research (page 15)

Q1 Firstly, as with any patient who has had recent diagnosis of cancer, Eshan will be apprehensive and frightened. It also appears that his healthcare to date has not been responsive to his religious and cultural needs – his preference for a nurse of the same gender for instance.

Q2 Eshan, as a Sikh, and an adherent Sikh will need to wear what is known as the 'five articles of faith' also called the 5 K's. The resources in the further reading section will enable you to read about these but, in terms of the recent MRI scan, the concern relates to the wearing of the Kara – an iron or steel bangle – and the Kirpan – a small sword or knife - which, as with all of the five articles of faith, must not be removed. There are other requirements such as the ability to pray at specific times in the day, access to free-flowing water to wash in and some dietary preferences – not accommodating these can cause significant distress.

Q3 A comprehensive assessment at the point of admission could and should identify all of Eshan's needs – all of his daily activities would be linked to his religious and cultural requirements and could easily be identified. Obviously, for this to be of any use, the assessment needs to underpin the plan of care including the need for any adjustments and this then has to be effectively communicated to all of the multi-disciplinary team who will care for Eshan.

Activity 1.7 Know the theory/Research (page 16)

One could argue that many of the specific platforms and proficiencies contained within both the Standards of Proficiency (NMC, 2024) and the Code (NMC, 2018) can be linked to the principles of assessment, planning and monitoring. However, some of the more obvious are provided as some examples below:

The Standards of Proficiency for Nursing Associates:

1.9 Communicate effectively using a range of skills and strategies with colleagues and people at all stages of life and with a range of mental, physical, cognitive, and behavioural health challenges.

1.10 Demonstrate the skills and abilities required to develop, manage, and maintain appropriate relationships with people, their families, carers, and colleagues.

1.11 Provide, promote, and where appropriate advocate for, nondiscriminatory, person-centred, and sensitive care at all times. Reflect on people's values and beliefs, diverse backgrounds, cultural characteristics, language requirements, needs, and preferences, taking account of any need for adjustments.

Pretty much all of Platform 3 but especially:

3.1 Demonstrate an understanding of human development from conception to death, to enable delivery of safe and effective person-centred care.

3.4 Demonstrate the knowledge, communication and relationship management skills required to provide people, families, and carers with accurate information that meets their needs before, during and after a range of interventions.

3.5 Work in partnership with people, to encourage shared decision-making, in order to support individuals, their families and carers to manage their own care when appropriate.

4.5 Demonstrate an ability to prioritise and manage their own workload, and recognise where elements of care can safely be delegated to other colleagues, carers, and family members.

The Code: Professional standards of practice and behaviour for nurses, midwives, and nursing associates:

2.1 Work in partnership with people to make sure you deliver care effectively.
2.2 Recognise and respect the contribution that people can make to their own health and well-being.
2.3 Encourage and empower people to share in decisions about their treatment and care.
6.1 Make sure that any information or advice given is evidence-based including information relating to using any health and care products or services.
13.1 Accurately identify, observe and assess signs of normal or worsening physical and mental health in the person receiving care.

Further reading

Factsheet: Key legislation and case law relating to decision-making and consent. Available at: www.gmc-uk.org/-/media/documents/factsheet—key-legislation-and-case-law-relating-to-decision-making-and-consent-84176182.pdf

This factsheet is provided by the General Medical Council (the doctors equivalent of the NMC), it is an accessible description of a number of cases that have had an impact on decision-making for all healthcare professionals.

Person-centred care made simple. What everyone should know about person-centred-care. Available at: www.health.org.uk/sites/default/files/PersonCentredCareMadeSimple.pdf

Religious Needs Resource, provided by Queens Court Hospice and therefore with sections relating to end of life care and care of the deceased, this also contains a free to access resource which highlights specific information about all major faiths. Available at: www.queenscourt.org.uk/resources-training/resource-library/religious-needs-resource/

NHS Education for Scotland guidelines for spiritual care – really useful guide to all of the major religions. Available at: www.nes.scot.nhs.uk/media/ay4je0io/multi-faith-resource-for-healthcare-staff.pdf.

Chapter 2

Working in partnership with people

Sarah Tobin

NMC *STANDARDS FOR PROFICIENCY FOR NURSING ASSOCIATES*

This chapter will address the following platforms and proficiencies:

Platform 1: Being an accountable practitioner

1.1   understand and act in accordance with the Code: Professional standards of practice and behaviour for nurses, midwives, and nursing associates, and fulfil all registration requirements.

1.10   demonstrate the skills and abilities required to develop, manage, and maintain appropriate relationships with people, their families, carers, and colleagues.

Platform 3: Provide and monitor care

3.5   work in partnership with people to encourage shared decision-making, in order to support individuals, their families and carers to manage their own care when appropriate.

Platform 4: Working in teams

4.1   demonstrate an awareness of the roles, responsibilities, and scope of practice of different members of the nursing and interdisciplinary team, and their own role within it.

Platform 6: Contributing to integrated care

6.1   understand the roles of the different providers of health and care. Demonstrate the ability to work collaboratively and in partnership with professionals from different agencies in inter-disciplinary teams.

Annexe A: Communication and relationship management skills

4. demonstrate effective communication skills for working in professional teams.

Introduction

As a registered nursing associate (RNA), you will have to provide compassionate, safe and effective care to adult, child, mental health and learning disabled patients and in a variety of settings. In order to do this, you will continually monitor the individual health needs of people within your care working in partnership with people, family, and carers. Student nursing associates (SNAs) and RNAs contribute to ongoing assessment and recognise when to refer to others within the wider multi-disciplinary team (MDT) for input and further assessment.

According to the Royal College of Nursing (RCN) in 2023, 'nursing is an ever growing and innovative profession and nurses are working in multi professional teams across health and care settings. Nurses are in a unique position to deliver care in partnership with people and carers, wherever care is needed'.

It is therefore evident that nursing, whilst a specialised and valuable profession within healthcare provision, cannot operate in isolation. The most crucial relationship is the one forged between the nursing associate and the person that they are caring for – the patient and their family. Much has been written about patient-centredness (a list of additional resources can be found at the end of this chapter), and it is an important response to care that previously had a more biomedical and disease-oriented approach. However, in order to ensure the person receives the care that they need they will require adequate, personalised assessments to identify what is best for them and this includes the need for other, specialised input.

Recent policy and guidance have emphasised the need for a more collaborative and joined-up approach to patient care and both emphasis and funding have been diverted in recent years to this end. No matter where you work, it will not be in isolation and all RNAs will need to have an understanding of how and why their assessment and subsequent patient care plan needs to include the input of all relevant professionals and services.

Personhood leads to person- and family-centred care

In Chapter 1, we described the importance of recognising the unique and dynamic nature of every single individual patient that you will encounter as an RNA. Without tailoring your care to that person, as much as is possible, there will be the risk that either the patient will not get the care they need or that they will not engage in the care provided. The way to ensure person-centred care is to assess each person as the individual that they are and in relation to the family and support that they live within.

Case study 2.1: Harry

Harry is 54 and has a mild learning disability, he works as an agricultural labourer and lives with his parents who are both in their early 80s. Harry was diagnosed as a Type II diabetic six years ago and is monitored and supported by the Practice Nurse Specialist at his local GP surgery, he also sees the podiatrist and has had input from the community dietician. These health professionals know Harry well, as does his GP who normally provides or coordinates an annual health check for Harry. They are aware that Harry cannot read so they always telephone him with his appointment details and, with his permission, tell his parents who put it on their calendar.

Harry was at work when he complained of pain in his chest, and he became rather clammy and pale – his colleagues called an ambulance. Harry was taken to hospital and, following tests, was diagnosed with angina. He was given a prescription for regular beta blockers, a statin, aspirin at low dose and given a GTN spray to use as required. He was discharged home with a follow-up OPA with the cardiology team in six weeks' time. A discharge summary was sent to the GP and was seen by a locum GP who added a note to Harry's records and updated his repeat prescription.

Harry did not fill the prescription nor take the beta blockers, statin, or aspirin and did not understand what the GTN spray was for, he returned to work the following day. He received a letter from the hospital with his OPA details but did not subsequently attend the appointment. Six months later Harry collapsed at work, he was taken to hospital where tests revealed he had suffered an acute MI, he was admitted to the CCU and subsequently underwent coronary artery stenting. His parents are very worried as their health is deteriorating and they relied on Harry to do much of the physically demanding work around the house, they are unsure if they will be able to cope in future.

Activity 2.1 Skill

Reading Harry's case study, it would seem that there may have been a lack of person-centred care; certainly, the patient failed to follow the planned care nor take the prescribed medication. Harry is unique and would very definitely have needed his care and treatment to be tailored to his specific needs.

Take a moment to list any specific assessments Harry needed and how this could have improved his plan of care.

Think of the resources and people that could have been used to support Harry and which do not seem to have been utilised.

A model answer is provided at the end of the chapter.

Person-centred care requires healthcare professionals to ensure that all of the resources, relevant experts, and support provision is provided to meet the needs of the individual. This is no easy task, to provide truly person-centred care also means providing joined-up care and this, in turn, requires effective communication, record keeping and coordination.

And, of course, the most important communication and the most important input is from the patient themselves. The statutory guidance from NHS England (2022, p. 7) highlights that *'involving people and communities is a legal requirement, working with them also supports the wider objectives of integration including population health management, personalisation of care and support, addressing health inequalities and improving quality'*. However, in his recent report (Department of Health and Social Care, 2024), Lord Darzi made it clear that more needs to be done; he states that the patient voice is not loud enough and that patients are now less empowered to make choices about their care.

Activity 2.2   Reflection

Think about your recent experience working in healthcare. What initiatives or processes were you aware of that sought the views, input and feedback from service users? Can you think of any and, if you can, what is the outcome of that process or initiative? If you do not know what happens with the feedback or how the engagement influences your organisation – what prevents you from having this understanding?

Finally, if you cannot recall any such schemes then imagine you have the ability to initiate a patient engagement project – what might work in your area of practice? What impact would you want to have?

As this is a reflective activity, no model answer is provided but some suggestions to support your ideas are given at the end of the chapter.

It would seem unarguable that patients need to be central to the care and the decisions about care that impact them. It also seems evident that this is not always the case – it is therefore a requirement of any assessment to fully establish the understanding and priorities of the patient. When working in partnership it is important to remember that the most important partnership is that formed between each patient and those, both individuals and organisations, who are responsible for providing care. It is also clear that patients often require more input than that provided by a single healthcare professional or team. It is therefore a requirement that effective care planning encompasses the need to refer to and liaise with the wider multi-disciplinary team.

We can't be all things to all people – why we need to refer to others

The Health Foundation (2023a) suggested that there will be significant change in the levels of demand and in the type of conditions people will need support for. The number of people in the UK living with major illness is expected to increase by a third – an extra 2.5 million people – by 2040. In addition, whilst there is a slowing down of the rate at which life expectancy increases it is still increasing – between 2018 and 2028 the number of people aged 75–84 is expected to increase by a third and those over 85 by a fifth. The report highlighted that people are living on average an additional 1.3 years with major illness compared with 2010 and that by 2040, 1 in 5 people will be living with a major illness. An assessment of the projected illness burden in England alone by 2040 suggests that, amongst others, the incidence of diabetes will increase by 49 per cent, dementia by 45 per cent, heart failure by 92 per cent and cancer by 31 per cent. With an ageing population and a more chronic burden of major illness the need to provide specialist, person-centred care is obvious.

Case study 2.2: Brenda

Imagine that you are an RNA working in an Emergency Medical Unit and have been asked to do the initial admission paperwork for a newly arrived patient who has been sent in by their GP via ambulance.

Brenda Stephens is a 72-year-old lady who was diagnosed with pancreatic cancer just over three months ago. Initially treated with chemotherapy this has been discontinued as the cancer progressed despite the treatment and Brenda found the burden of side-effects too difficult to tolerate. The MDT decision made along with Brenda and her close family is to opt for symptom management to optimise Brenda's quality of life. On admission, Brenda is clearly jaundiced, is complaining of extreme itching of her skin, is nauseated and reports she is eating little, she has some pain which is mostly in her back and which scores 3/10 on an analogue pain scale.

The reason for admission is that her left lower leg has become swollen and the calf painful to touch – the GP is concerned that she may have a deep-vein thrombosis (DVT) and wants this confirmed or excluded. The GP letter requests that Brenda is detained in hospital for as little time as possible as she is keen to return home to her husband and family as soon as possible. Brenda undergoes an ultrasound test which confirms that she has a DVT in her popliteal vein. The on-call medical team prescribes once daily low molecular weight heparin injections and an oral Xa inhibitor medication. The initial doses of both drugs are given in hospital, the medications are dispensed, and Brenda is discharged home.

Activity 2.3   Critical thinking

Read Brenda's case study and take a moment to consider all of the potential services and specialist input that has and will be supporting Brenda in the months since she was diagnosed. Make a list of everything you think of.

Once you have compiled this list, consider who or what services will still be involved with her and her family's care.

Finally, decide whether any new service/support will be needed following the new diagnosis and who you may need to liaise with prior to discharging Brenda home.

A model answer is provided at the end of this chapter.

Activity 2.3 should highlight the need for the input of multiple resources to ensure that Brenda gets the best, most effective care based on her assessed needs and the requirement for this to be coordinated. And that all sounds very straightforward. However, there are many reasons why it is not always easy and sometimes not even possible to provide what is needed for every patient. This will be discussed more fully later in this chapter and in Chapter 7, but one area that is readily acknowledged as causing challenge and inequality in service access and provision is the impact of deprivation.

An initiative by the NHS (2021) known as the National Healthcare Inequalities Improvement Programme was established to work with existing programmes and policy across the NHS in England, amongst other systems, to deliver exceptional healthcare for all in terms of access, experience, and outcomes. Health inequalities are defined as unequal and avoidable differences in health across the population and within different groups in society. One determinant of how likely you are to receive unfair access and/or treatment is the level of deprivation you experience as evidence demonstrates that those who live in the most deprived areas face the worst inequalities.

Activity 2.4   Research

Using your preferred online Search Engine search for 'National Healthcare Inequalities Improvement Programme'. Once on the site navigate through the sections (index can be found on the right-hand side of the homepage) to the 'Deprivation' section.

List the seven different factors that combine to form the index of deprivation.

Then scroll down and look at the 'Core20PLUS5' initiative which seeks to support the most deprived 20 per cent of the national population – what other groups are listed as often impacted by deprivation?

A model answer is included at the end of this chapter.

Subsequent chapters will look specifically at the some of these issues in greater depth, but you will need to consider health inequalities and deprivation in relation to accessing support for those you plan and provide care for. Think about the case study earlier in this chapter – Harry is 54 and experiencing significant health issues. This is not unexpected, the average life expectancy for a man in England (with slight variations in the other UK nations) is 79.1 years (Office of National Statistics, 2024). According to the latest Learning Disability Mortality Review (LeDeR, 2022), the median age of death for a person with a learning disability is 63 – a significant difference when compared with the general population. Worryingly, the average age of death in those who have a learning disability and are also from Black, South Asian, or other minority ethnic backgrounds is 34 years (NHS, 2023).

There are many reasons that may explain these discrepancies, some suggested include lack of understanding of learning disability from healthcare professionals, lack of access to transport, to finance, to accessible information about healthcare and choices, communication issues, increased prevalence of underlying health conditions and an overall higher incidence of deprivation in these populations. Whatever the reason, it would be important for these issues to be considered when assessing need or formulating a plan of care. Without acknowledging the wider challenges a person faces, a plan of care may well fail – Harry demonstrates this very clearly.

The importance of care coordination

If one accepts that more than one individual or team frequently needs to be involved in a person's care then, equally, one must accept the need for coordination of that care. It is clear that poor coordination and inadequate communication results in added complexity for patients and care teams and may result in poorer outcomes for patients.

Multi-disciplinary teams (MDT)

The World Health Organization (2022) noted the importance of effectively working together and stated that the 'establishment of teamwork and collaboration in multi-professional teams is a major skill-mix change and is key for organising and coordinating health and care services'. So, what is a multi-professional or multi-disciplinary team (MDT)? The concept of an MDT is not new but in recent years greater emphasis has been placed on promoting MDT working. Perhaps most impactful, the *NHS Long Term Plan* in 2019 set out to break down barriers between teams and organisations, an ambition further highlighted in *We are the NHS: People Plan 2020/21*.

Health Education England (2021) suggests that an MDT is a team 'consisting of individuals drawn from different disciplines who come together to achieve a common goal'. The Social Care Institute for Excellence (2024) identified the key components of an MDT as follows:

- An identified manager or practice leader responsible for facilitating the team's overall function.
- Joint meetings to share insights and concerns.
- A shared digital record of all contacts.
- Assessments and interventions of team members with an individual and their family.
- A key worker system established, coordinating care for those with complex support packages under the guidance of a named team member.
- The team composition reflects the diversity of professions and disciplines, ensuring alignment with the needs of the target population.

As an example of MDT working, an RNA working in a mental health in-patient unit notices that the service user they are admitting has several, additional issues. The service user states that they do not really understand the new medication that they have recently started and also that they have a poor appetite and have lost some weight recently. Having admitted the service user, the RNA contacts the unit pharmacist and asks if they can come and see the newly admitted service user and also sends a referral requesting review by the mental health service dietician. The RNA also ensures that these concerns are accurately recorded in the relevant paperwork and that the service user's key worker is informed of the referrals.

MDTs can work in all areas and across the boundaries between primary and secondary care and between statutory services and those provided by the private or voluntary sector if necessary. A common approach is the development of community-based MDTs, in which a mix of health and care professionals come together to plan and coordinate people's care. Many MDTs are based around general practices and typically focus on care for adults with complex health and care needs (Health Foundation, 2023b).

The key to MDT working is that it does not work in isolation – an MDT that does not encompass or access the relevant resources and personnel will risk being inefficient and ineffective. The aim of an MDT approach is the opposite of 'silo' working, so needs to ensure that mechanisms exist to cross boundaries – perceived and physical – because that is how patients should and do receive care.

Interprofessional care

One aspect of interprofessional working, the MDT approach described above, can help to ensure a range of expertise, and perspectives are available to help support patient care, but often MDTs exist within specific services and organisations. Take, for example, the colorectal cancer MDT (the National Cancer Plan in 2000 mandated that all cancer patients receive care from MDTs), this MDT will generally comprise healthcare staff from a variety of professions – doctors (gastroenterologist, oncologist, and palliative care), nurses (colorectal clinical nurse specialist, stoma nurse specialist), surgeons, pathologists, radiologists, and dieticians. The decision that they will make about the best possible treatment plan for a patient is undeniably enhanced by having a body of expert assessment and knowledge to inform it. However, this MDT is comprised of experts in colorectal cancer and a patient who presents with this may well have other health conditions or face additional challenges in terms of the level of deprivation they live with.

In the model of care described above, the MDT will undoubtedly recommend excellent care to address the patient's colorectal cancer, but what if they also have Parkinson's disease or any number of other long-term conditions? Unless all aspects of their health needs are addressed collaboratively it is likely that the excellent cancer care will be less effective or not even possible if their other health needs are not also assessed and optimised. This is where **interprofessional** liaison and care is important – the MDT will need to liaise with the patient's General Practitioner, the clinical team managing their Parkinson's disease and perhaps contact staff in primary and social care if the patient has increased need for care and support. Not providing such interprofessional care is a little like ensuring that your car has adequate fuel and oil but not pumping up flat tyres and then being surprised when you can't drive away in it! Excellent care in one area is undermined by lack of equally well-managed care in another.

Activity 2.5   Reflection

In Activity 2.1, you were asked to make a list of what resources and people could have been used to help support the plan of care for Harry.

Return to that list again, but this time think about where those people are based, or perhaps need to be based. If all of those people provide 'their' expert care to Harry but this is done in isolation (as in silo working) what are the risks to both Harry and to service provision? How could assessments and plans be shared and how can we ensure care is 'joined-up'? Think about areas where you have worked – what initiatives, process and guidelines have you witnessed that could help?

As this is a reflective exercise no model answer is provided, but hints and ideas are available throughout this chapter and the book as a whole.

Interagency care

Whilst interprofessional care refers to the collaborative efforts of individual healthcare professionals from different disciplines, interagency care focuses on collaboration between different organisations. These organisations could be NHS services, local councils, police forces, charities, schools or housing, and environmental services. So, interprofessional care may be an RNA discussing a patient's care plan with a physiotherapist and with a community nurse and dietician whereas interagency care might be a local council working with the NHS to ensure a patient has suitable accommodation post discharge from hospital.

As with all aspects of integrated working, there are challenges and barriers that can make this difficult and overly complex to achieve. These include limited awareness of interprofessional roles, poor communication, different IT systems, hierarchies and different cultures, lack of time, misunderstandings about confidentiality, different funding streams and lack of training in interagency resources and interfaces.

However, a number of well-publicised and tragic cases highlighted the importance of ensuring effective interagency working. Following the death from malnutrition of a 40-year-old woman in a city in the Southwest of England, a safeguarding review highlighted the number of different organisations and agencies that were involved in her care. The review highlighted that the Mental Health services that were involved with her had a 'culture of avoiding consulting with the local safeguarding team'. Neighbours who were concerned for her welfare had contacted the police, the housing provider who was unaware that she was vulnerable had cut off her gas supply, she had out-patient appointments with a psychiatrist and other doctors, an ambulance crew attended her address. Many of these professionals noted her vulnerability, but little could be identified in terms of a cohesive plan of care. The safeguarding review concluded that the agencies involved in this woman's care 'worked very separately and shared no information' (Turner, 2017).

The awareness of the potential for harm when multiple agencies are involved in a person's care is very much evident when that care is provided to vulnerable children. Some cases, such as those of Peter Connelly (known as 'Baby P'), Victoria Climbié, Alfie Steele and Star Hobson are examples of those that receive significant media coverage. These are, unfortunately, only some examples of many more cases the majority of which do not achieve the same attention. The common factor in many cases is that the children harmed and even murdered are often known to multiple agencies – schools, social services, healthcare teams, the police as well as charitable organisations. The government's own statutory guidelines – *Working Together to Safeguard Children* (2023) – highlights that it is a guide to 'multi-agency working to help, protect and promote the welfare of children' which illustrates that a multi-agency approach is core to planning safe and effective care for children. And, as previously described, the pressures on families due to health inequalities and deprivation increases the risks. The children's charity Barnardo's published a report in 2024 which highlights that the cost-of-living crisis and the Covid-19 pandemic had worsened inequalities in society and that 4.2 million children were living in relative poverty in the UK (relative poverty is defined as households 60 per cent below the median average income after housing costs).

It is very evident that when assessing need and planning care for any vulnerable person and especially children, agencies need to communicate, cooperate, and consolidate their endeavours. And, whilst it is much easier to find reports and discussion about care that has failed it is evident that when care is coordinated the possibilities for a positive and sustainable outcomes are clear. One safeguarding partnership in the Northwest of England publish case studies highlighting successful multi-agency working and the significant impact this can have (see link in the further reading section if you need to read some positive stories).

Case study 2.3: Shahida

Shahida, aged 19, attends her local GP surgery as she has been complaining of severe headaches, she is accompanied by her mother. At Shahida's mother's request a chaperone, an RNA working at the surgery, also attends the consultation. During their discussion, the GP becomes concerned that there may be more to her symptoms than Shahida is disclosing – the GP suggests that they move to another room so that he might weigh Shahida. Once alone with the GP and RNA Shahida bursts into tears and explains that her parents are imminently taking her to Pakistan for an arranged marriage with a man she has never met. Shahida has a boyfriend but has not told her parents this, she says she loves her boyfriend and wants to leave and set up home with him. Shahida states that she is in fear for her safety if she does not do as her family dictates – at this point her mother enters the room looking for her.

Activity 2.6   Research

Read Shahida's fictitious scenario.

Do you consider it the responsibility of the doctor and RNA to take any action? Do they owe a duty of care to Shahida beyond addressing her presenting complaint of headaches?

Look at the NMC Code of Conduct and highlight any sections that would inform your decision.

Having made your decision and if you do need to help Shahida, what agencies would you need to liaise with to provide the necessary support and to ensure her safety?

A model answer is provided at the end of the chapter.

What is meant by integrated care?

It is clear that there are a number of different terms and descriptions for working in partnership with others and, where there are multiple terms and concepts, there is the potential for confusion. So, what does 'integrated care' mean and how is this different from any of the terms such as interagency or multi-disciplinary care discussed earlier? In 2022, the Health and Care Act set out to introduce new measures with the aim of making it simpler for all health and care providers to provide joined-up care for people and especially those who rely on several different services. The Act recognises that there are many more people living to a greater age and that these people may well have multiple health conditions that require input and ongoing support from various providers. One way to address this has been to set up Integrated Care Systems with the aim to bring all local services that fund and support patients together – not just within the NHS but also local authorities (councils or boroughs), charities and patient groups. Cutting down on 'red tape', simplifying processes, avoiding repetition and ensuring meaningful communication across departments and organisations aims to help make patient care more effective and more efficient. So, how is this different from the similar sounding 'interagency' care? Integrated care aims to go beyond ensuring effective communication and information sharing between teams by providing coordinated care pathways across different agencies with the aim of unifying patient experience with seamless transitions between different services.

Interprofessional and interagency care can be hampered, as described earlier in the chapter, by differences in working practice, different IT systems, different funding streams and so on. By integrating the patient pathway, the aim is to reduce inefficiency, reduce duplication and simplify care provision. For more information about integrated care systems and how the work please see the Kings Fund resource in the additional reading section at the end of the chapter.

Importantly, there cannot be integrated care without adequate and appropriate needs assessment to inform the appropriate plan of care and how and by whom this can be provided. The Social Care Institute for Excellence (2021) provided guidance that suggested that there needs to be 'joint needs assessment and care planning' to achieve integrated care. They state the following:

'In the past, individuals and their families were asked to undergo assessments of their health and/or social care needs by each professional who became involved. Whilst some aspects of such assessments may have differed due to the specialist nature of the service

and treatment on offer, much was in fact similar across all professionals. This meant that the individual had to repeat their details and stories on multiple occasions which took up much of their time, could unnecessarily delay access to support, and could require the sharing of personal and distressing information to numerous people. Professionals then used these assessments to develop their own care plans which did not sufficiently connect with and co-ordinate across those developed by other professionals.

The introduction of joint needs assessments and joined up plans of care could and should ensure that where information is common across different care environments there would no longer be the need for repetitive information sharing. More importantly, joint assessment and planning would ensure a cohesive and collaborative approach which included the patient and their family.

So, whether you aim to deliver interprofessional, interagency, or integrated care the beginning of the process will always be an effective assessment with the patient at the heart of the process. As a SNA or RNA, you are integral to this process as your skill and understanding will be used to inform and enhance this assessment and underpin any subsequent plan of care.

Inclusivity, civility, and compassion

This chapter has aimed to explain the importance of and mechanisms to ensure patient care is planned and delivered in partnership – with other healthcare providers and especially with the patient at the heart of the process. However, no approach or method to underpin this ambition can be foolproof – no approach can work for all people, all of the time. This is why being a registered professional is such a rewarding occupation – your judgement and knowledge will enable you to make appropriate clinical decisions, to use your critical thinking and reasoning skills. As such, having an understanding that some groups of people will always need additional help or a modified approach to their needs is crucial.

Studies by various charities and non-governmental organisations, as well as official data collection, highlights that care is not equal in this country (or, indeed across the world). Resource needs to be allocated fairly, and waste eliminated wherever possible to ensure maximum benefit to the end service user. Beauchamp and Childress (2019) suggest that taking an ethical approach to healthcare is necessary and that this can be achieved by ensuring care is based on the autonomous choice of the patient, aims to provide benefit (beneficence) whilst causing the least amount of harm (non-maleficence) and is a just (fair) resource. We know that this is not always the case – marginalised groups such as prisoners, the homeless, asylum seekers, those who do not speak English or cannot read English or those who live in poverty amongst others have demonstrably poorer health outcomes. Without the will to provide focused and personalised assessment for these groups there cannot be effective care provision, and such provision will often require integrated care approaches. The increase in long-term health conditions adds further complexity to this equation – again, the answer is assessment and integration. And, this does need to be considered and planned for; as mentioned earlier, the Health Foundation (2024) suggests that by 2040, 1 in 5 adults (around 9.3 million people) could be living with a major illness.

Inclusivity is important – whether ensuring that marginalised groups get fair and effective care or ensuring input from care providers from any necessary specialty or organisation. There is also increasing research and interests in the concepts of civility and compassion and the impact both of these can have on the outcomes of healthcare provision. The idea that 'civility saves lives' may seem far-fetched, but evidence suggests that incivility – rudeness and lack of kindness – significantly impacts on team performance and therefore the safety of care provided. Both this concept and the impact of compassion will be covered more fully in the final chapter of this book, but remember in Chapter 1 we stated that the root of the word 'assessment' comes from the Latin 'assidere' meaning to sit beside. In order to work in partnership with patients, their families and loved ones we need to treat them with compassion and sit beside them. In order to ensure integrated care in all its forms we need to sit with our colleagues, show them civility, listen to them, and understand their input.

Conclusion

Care that does not include the patient right from the very beginning, from the point of assessing need, will be more likely to fail, result in mistakes and risk wasting time and resources. Partnerships must exist between the patient and the caregiving team but also between relevant professionals, teams and organisations that provide care. The best and most effective care is delivered in this integrated and inclusive way. This idea is not new, in 2014 the Five Year Forward View set out a vision of a more integrated health and social care service, the 2019 NHS Long Term Plan set out further steps and a white paper in 2021 began the legislative changes needed to embed integration in England. However, there is no cause for complacency, despite the 2022 Health and Care Act which progressed this even further it is evident that poor integration remains a problem and especially so for those in marginalised groups. Medical advances and increasing life expectancy are successes to be celebrated but also need to be considered in terms of increased demand and greater complexity. Lack of resources in all areas of healthcare threaten progress to deliver effective, joined-up care. Thankfully, one approach to ensuring effective partnership working – that of civility and compassion – results in no monetary costs pressures and little in terms of resources.

Health inequalities, whilst evident and potentially growing, do not need to be seen as inevitable. With effective and appropriately mandated resources integrated care inequalities can be addressed. The greatest resource of all is the expert in each person's needs assessment and subsequent plan of care – the patient.

Chapter summary

This chapter has highlighted the role of the SNA or RNA in working in partnership with patients and other professionals in order to ensure the best possible care for each, unique person. The importance of understanding the role of and liaising with local MDTs and well as interprofessional and interagency referral has been described. The idea that one approach cannot work for all is considered and the need to understand that some groups of people require greater input and more complex care coordination. Finally, the idea that working in partnership requires care that is inclusive as well as being provided with compassion and civility completed the chapter.

Activities: Brief outline answers

Activity 2.1 Skill (page 25)

In relation to Harry's care: list any specific assessments Harry needed and how this could have improved his plan of care. Also, think of the resources and people that could have been used to support Harry and which do not seem to have been utilised.

- Capacity – Harry needed a capacity assessment as per the Mental Capacity Act 2005, this would determine whether he had the capacity to understand and consent to any proposed treatment. It would also highlight any deficits in his understanding.

- Communication – Harry needed an assessment to determine his preferred way of communicating and the need for any support or communication aids.
- Hospital passport – does Harry have hospital passport (a document about Harry and any specific needs) – if not, start one!

People in hospital:

1. Learning Disability Nurse Specialist
2. Speech and Language Therapist – can provide communication aids
3. Discharge liaison team
4. Outreach cardiology team if available

People in the community:

1. General Practitioner – usual discharge summary was not adequate, needed direct contact
2. Community Learning Disability Team
3. Community Nurse
4. Community dietician

This is not an exhaustive list but starts to demonstrate how many people and what resource could have been available to Harry, any one of which could have prevented the breakdown in his care.

Activity 2.2 Reflection (page 26)

Some ideas to help with this reflective activity – nationally the NHS has the 'Friends and Family' test which provides a quick and anonymous way to provide feedback after receiving NHS care and treatment. The platform 'Care Opinion' allows people to provide publicly accessible feedback about their care.

Many NHS organisations (including the NHS itself) have a website or social media platform where you can leave feedback.

Formal complaints are collated and can provide the basis for learning and improvement – all organisations have a mechanism to handle complaints.

On a more local level individual departments, units or organisations can produce surveys and audits, can provide suggestion boxes and display feedback in patient areas.

Local 'working with us' or 'patient panels' can be set up to ensure service users can provide direct input into service development and improvement.

Activity 2.3 Critical thinking (page 27)

Some examples of the services and specialists Brenda could have had access to since her diagnosis include:

- General Practitioner
- Gastroenterologist
- Endoscopy unit and staff
- Upper Gastrointestinal (GI) Clinical Nurse Specialist (CNS)

- Upper GI Cancer MDT – multiple staff members
- Oncologist
- Chemotherapy staff and CNS
- Dietician
- Palliative Care Team
- Occupational Therapist
- Community Nursing Team
- Social Care Team
- Psychologist

Those underlined may still be in contact with Brenda.

Since Brenda has been newly diagnosed with a DVT it will be important for those members of the interprofessional and interagency teams to be made aware of this change in her care.

Activity 2.4 Research (page 28)

The index of multiple deprivation ranks each small area in England from most to least deprived based on a combination of seven different factors including:

- Income
- Employment
- Education
- Health
- Crime
- Barriers to housing and services
- Living environment

Groups identified as being more vulnerable to health inequalities include:

- Ethnic minority communities
- People with Learning Disability including autism
- Those with multiple long-term conditions
- Those with protected characteristics as defined by the Equality Act 2010.
- The homeless
- Those with drug and alcohol dependence
- Vulnerable migrants
- Gypsy, Roma and Traveller communities
- Sex workers
- People in contact with the justice system
- Victims of modern slavery
- Other socially excluded groups.

Activity 2.6 Research (page 32)

The GP and the RNA are both responsible for ensuring Shahida's safety – both act within the standards that are mandated by their individual regulatory bodies – for the GP that is the General Medical Council and for the RNA it is the Nursing and Midwifery Council. Both of these organisations make it clear that Shahida is owed a duty of care as expected from the 'ordinarily competent practitioner'.

The NMC Code states that in relation to patients, Registered nurses should 'make their care and safety your main concern'. And *16.1 raise and, if necessary, escalate any concerns you may have about patient or public safety, or the level of care people are receiving in your workplace or any other health and care setting and use the channels available to you in line with our guidance and your local working practices. And 17.1 take all reasonable steps to protect people who are vulnerable or at risk from harm, neglect, or abuse.* Both individuals must also act within the law and forced marriage is illegal in England and Wales.

Those who you could liaise with include:

- Forced Marriage Unit – a government organisation that can provide advice, find a safe place to stay, and impact visas for travel abroad.
- The local Safeguarding team
- The police
- Domestic abuse and forced marriage helpline (in Scotland)
- Charitable organisations such as Karma Nirvana, Freedom Charity, the Halo Project
- Refuge – provide a 24-hour helpline and can help with safe places to stay
- Local religious or cultural centres that may be able to provide support to Shahida and/or her family.

Further reading

Harris, M. (2024) *Understanding Person-Centred Care for Nursing Associates* (2nd edition). Sage: London.

This is another book in the UNAP series which complements some of the points in this chapter relating to the link between partnership working and the provision of person-centred care.

Kelsall-Knight, L. and Stevens, R. (2023) Exploring the implementation of person-centred care in nursing practice. *Nursing Standard* doi: 10.7748/ns.2023.e12190

This is a clear and straightforward article explaining person-centred care as well as what can be done to support it and how we might remove barriers to it, also includes a lot of useful references that can be followed up for even more information.

The Kings Fund. (2022) Integrated care systems explained: Making sense of systems, places and neighbourhoods. Available at: www.kingsfund.org.uk/insight-and-analysis/long-reads/integrated-care-systems-explained

Integrated care systems are mentioned a number of times in this chapter – this resource from the Kings Fund explains what they are, how they work and provides an integrated map so you can discover more about the impact in your local area.

Wirral Safeguarding Children Partnership Annual Report 2021 on Multi-agency working. Available at: www.wirralsafeguarding.co.uk/annual-report-2021-multi-agency-working/ for some positive case studies highlighting the impact of muti-agency working.

Chapter 3

Bio-psycho-social healthcare assessment

Lisa-Marie Rowe

NMC *STANDARDS FOR PROFICIENCY FOR NURSING ASSOCIATES*

This chapter will address the following platforms and proficiencies:

Platform 1: Being an accountable practitioner

1.1 understand and act in accordance with the Code: Professional standards of practice and behaviour for nurses, midwives, and nursing associates, and fulfil all registration requirements.

1.11 reflect on people's values and beliefs, diverse backgrounds, cultural characteristics, language requirements, needs, and preferences, taking account of any need for adjustments.

Platform 2: Promoting health and preventing ill health

2.6 understand and explain the contribution of social influences, health literacy, individual circumstances, behaviours, and lifestyle choices to mental, physical, and behavioural health outcomes.

Platform 3: Provide and monitor care

3.3 recognise and apply knowledge of commonly encountered mental, physical, behavioural, and cognitive health conditions when delivering care.

3.19 demonstrate an understanding of co-morbidities and the demands of meeting people's holistic needs when prioritising care.

Platform 6: Contributing to integrated care

6.1 understand the roles of the different providers of health and care. Demonstrate the ability to work collaboratively and in partnership with professionals from different agencies in interdisciplinary teams.

6.2 understand and explore the challenges of providing safe nursing care for people with complex co-morbidities and complex care needs.

6.3 demonstrate an understanding of the complexities of providing mental, cognitive, behavioural, and physical care needs across a wide range of integrated care settings.

Chapter aims

After reading this chapter you will:

- Be able to explain the theory and principles of the bio-psycho-social model.
- Understand how a person's bio-psycho-social needs can affect one another.
- Understand how the bio-psycho-social model supports a person-centred approach.
- Recognise the importance of inter-disciplinary working to meet the bio-psycho-social needs of an individual.

Introduction

This chapter will explore how an individual's biological, psychological and social needs are intertwined and affect a person's overall health and well-being.

It will encourage the reader to consider the impact of different needs upon one another and how this affects the delivery of care. It will explain how the bio-psycho-social model emerged over time and how the model can be used within all specialities of nursing to deliver person-centred care.

Historical overview

For centuries, clinicians disregarded the influence of psychological and sociological factors upon health. It was considered that poor health was caused by a biological fault rather than the result of psychological and social factors such as poor living conditions for example. The emphasis was on diagnosing and treating an illness rather than treating a person based upon their individual state of health and well-being.

In 1942, the Beveridge report was presented to parliament. The report aimed to eradicate the five 'Great Evils' which were said to plague society: Want, Disease, Ignorance, Squalor, and Idleness. Although not implemented until after the Second World War the report led to the introduction of:

- A social security system which acted as a safety net for those who were elderly, unwell, or on maternity leave;
- The introduction of the National Health Service (NHS) which was to be free at the point of delivery to all;
- Improved access to education, including adult education;
- Improved living conditions through the building of council housing;
- The creation of more jobs.

The formation of the Welfare State was celebrated as accessible to all from 'cradle to the grave'. Beveridge was approaching welfare by tackling both the physical and the social needs of the population and moving away from the biomedical approach.

In 1977, Engel wrote about the correlation between an individual's biological, psychological, and social (BPS) needs. Engel's BPS model (see Figure 3.1) moved away from ritualised or paternalistic care and towards patient-centred care where it was recognised that biological, social, and psychological factors all affect one another and a person's overall health and well-being. This emphasised a more holistic approach to health rather than a biomedical approach to illness.

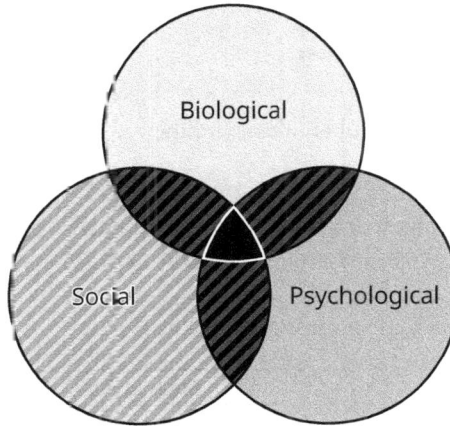

Figure 3.1   The bio-psycho-social (BPS) model (Engel, 1977)

The BPS model states that multiple factors produce multiple effects upon a person's health. A definition of health provided by the World Health Organization (WHO) Constitution (2024) states: 'Health is a state of complete physical, mental, and social well-being and not merely the absence of disease or infirmity'.

Activity 3.1   Reflection

Consider when you have felt unwell.

- What were your physical symptoms?
- How did it make you feel psychologically?
- How did being unwell affect you socially?
- What made you feel better?

It is likely that medication was not the only method of making you feel better.

As this activity is based on your own observation, there is no outline answer at the end of the chapter.

The BPS model provides a humanistic approach whereby no person's illness is reduced to one contributory factor. It allows healthcare professionals to obtain a clear picture of an individual and what is important to them. The BPS model encourages healthcare professionals to consider an individual's circumstances and the impact of these upon their overall health. In turn this aids diagnosis as the patient relays information which could provide details of contributing factors to their ill health. Therefore, we need to recognise the person as a whole-being. This is known as holism.

Housing

Housing is a clear example of how social status can affect biological and psychological health. Poor housing can affect people in several ways:

- Respiratory conditions such as Asthma
- Cardiovascular conditions
- An increase in accidental injury
- Mental Health conditions
- Overcrowding
- Infectious diseases including tuberculosis, influenza, and diarrhoea.

The World Health Organization (2018).

Equally, where a person lives can affect them biologically, psychologically, and socially. Table 3.1 shows some differences between urban and rural areas.

Table 3.1   Differences between urban and rural areas

Urban area	Rural area
High density population	Low density population
Access to public transport	Poor/infrequent public transport
Easy access to shops and supermarkets	Limited access to shops and supermarkets
Limited green space	Access to green space
Inhalation of fumes/pollution	Cleaner air
Access to specialised health care	Sense of community
Greater employability opportunities	Fewer job opportunities

Case study 3.1: Joan Part 1

Joan is 74 years old and lives in a cottage in a very rural area. She is recently widowed and has type 2 diabetes, hypertension, and osteoarthritis. Her husband used to drive so they could access their groceries, the doctors, chemist and attend Church. This was especially useful as the nearest shop is a 15-minute drive away. Since she has been living alone; her daughter has set up a supermarket delivery for her mum. As Joan finds it hard to stand for long periods to cook, they have ordered frozen microwave meals.

Activity 3.2   Critical thinking

Joan's bio-psycho-social needs have been separated in the list above. However, these do affect one another.

Draw and add the needs into the BPS model from Figure 3.1. How do they affect each other? For example, you may identify how Joan's diet may affect her hypertension and type 2 diabetes.

Biopsychosocial model: Joan's needs

Biological needs (The 'bio' circle) These factors relate to Joan's physical health, genetics and bodily functions.

Type 2 diabetes, Osteoarthritis and Hypertension: These chronic conditions require ongoing monitoring, medication management and a controlled diet.

Psychological needs (The 'psycho' circle): These factors encompass Joan's mental health, emotions and coping mechanisms.

- **Grief:** As a recent widow, she is dealing with the emotional and mental toll of losing her husband.
- **Coping with change:** She must adapt to a new lifestyle that includes living alone and experiencing loneliness.

Social needs (The 'social' circle): These factors include Joan's social environment, relationships and external circumstances.

- **Social isolation:** Her rural location and inability to drive mean she is cut off from her community, including her church and social network.
- **Lack of transportation:** The loss of her husband's driving means she can no longer access services or social outings on her own.
- **Loss of a caregiver:** Her husband was a critical support system, and his absence leaves a major gap in her daily care and companionships.

Joan's bio-psycho-social needs can be separated as follows:

Biological needs:

- Type 2 diabetes
- Hypertension
- Osteoarthritis

Psychological needs:

- Recently widowed
- Daughter lives far away
- Pain from osteoarthritis

Social needs:

- Socially isolated – difficulty in accessing doctors, chemist and Church
- Groceries delivered weekly (ready meals have high salt and sugar content).

Intersections of needs (The overlapping sections)

Joan's situation demonstrates how these domains do not exist in isolation but constantly influence each other.

Biological and social overlap

- **Groceries:** Her rural location (social) combined with her limited mobility and health issues (biological) prevent her from driving to get groceries. This is mitigated by her daughter arranging delivery, but it is a direct result of the intersection of her needs.

(Continued)

- **Healthcare access:** Her physical conditions (biological) are managed in a more challenging way due to her remote location and lack of transport (social), requiring arrangements for chemist and doctor visits.
- **Dietary needs:** The inability to easily get fresh groceries (social) can impact her ability to manage her diabetes through diet (biological).
- **Reduced mobility:** The physical effects of her conditions limit her ability to perform daily tasks and leave her home.
- **Cardiovascular risks:** Long-term social isolation and loneliness are associated with a higher risk of heart disease, high blood pressure and stroke. Inflammation promoted by isolation can accelerate the buildup of plaque in arteries.

Biological and psychological overlap

Cooking difficulty: Osteoarthritis pain (biological) makes it hard for her to cook for long periods, which can lead to stress and frustration (psychological).

Illness and grief: The stress of grieving (psychological) can worsen her physical health conditions, such as hypertension (biological). The isolation and grief can also make it harder for her to manage her diabetes effectively.

Weakened immune function: Chronic stress and elevated inflammation can suppress immune system function link to diabetes also.

Psychological and social overlap

- **Grief:** Companionship and support from family and social connections is recognised to help people in the grieving process.
- **Mental health disorders:** Social isolation is both a risk factor for and a consequence of mental health issues. It is strongly linked with increased rates of anxiety, depression and post-traumatic stress disorder (PTSD).

Biological, psychological and social overlap

Holistic well-being: The combined effect of all these factors on Joan's overall well-being is clear. The death of her husband created social isolation and grief (social and psychological), which affects her ability to manage her chronic health conditions (biological). The solutions, like food delivery from her daughter, help manage the logistical social needs but don't fully address the mental or physical challenges.

Type two diabetes can affect all BPS needs including stress, anxiety and depression, social stigma, poor social-economic status, age, genetics, obesity and other comorbidities. For example, Joan's poor mobility due to pain will affect her ability to exercise and to maintain a healthy weight.

- Hypertension: biopsychosocial considerations for hypertension include biological factors like genetics, hormone imbalances and physiological responses to stress, which can elevate blood pressure. Social isolation is a psychological stressor that affects hypertension by activating the sympathetic nervous system. An increase in the stress hormone cortisol can damage tissues and increase inflammation over time.

The bio-psycho-social model and person-centred care

The BPS model is closely aligned to person-centred care. Person-centred care relies on effective communication and creating a therapeutic relationship. Once a therapeutic relationship is established, the healthcare professional can find out about the person's individual needs and preferences. A nursing associate is expected to 'work in partnership with people, to encourage shared decision-making, in order to support individuals, their families and carers to manage their own care when appropriate' (NMC, 2018).

Delivering person-centred care also encourages autonomy and the person's right to self-determination. Working in partnership with people 'creates better patient outcomes and costs less to health and care systems' (NHS England, 2024). Person-centred care also encourages people to take responsibility to maintain and improve their health. Rather than care being provided for them or done to them, they are in control and central to all decision-making – a concept supported in 'no decision about me, without me' (Coulter and Collins, 2011).

What is important to a person and what they prioritise can be different to factors prioritised by healthcare professionals. The NHS Long Term Plan (2019) recognised this and aimed for people to have autonomy and control over their own individual care. Healthcare professionals must respect a person's ability to make unwise decisions (MCA, 2005) and record a person's decisions and choices – 'write accurate, clear, legible records and documentation' (NMC, 2018).

Barriers to implementing person-centred care include:

- Fears of litigation;
- Accountability;
- The ability of staff to make decisions regarding capacity;
- Patients being labelled as 'non-compliant';
- Time;
- Communication difficulties;
- Power imbalances;
- Institutionalisation.

Protected characteristics and the bio-psycho-social model

Person-centred care must consider protected characteristics, a person's views and wishes and how these may impact upon care provision. Nursing associates are required to:

1.11 *Reflect on people's values and beliefs, diverse backgrounds, cultural characteristics, language requirements, needs and preferences, taking account of any need for adjustments* (NMC, 2018).

Under the Equality Act (2010) it is unlawful to discriminate against someone because of a protected characteristic. The Act specifies that the advancement of equality relies upon:

- Removing or minimising disadvantage suffered by people due to their protected characteristics;
- Taking steps to meet the needs of people from protected groups where these are different from the needs of other people;

- Encouraging people from protected groups to participate in public life or in activities where their participation is disproportionately low.

Therefore, it is important to recognise that those with protected characteristics are generally more likely to experience specific BPS needs. Some examples are provided below.

- Age – older persons are more likely to experience multi-co-morbidities, be socially isolated and experience loneliness.
- Disability – people with a disability may find difficulties in accessing services, there may be poor public transport provision and barriers to employment.
- Gender reassignment – there is a higher prevalence of anxiety and depression in persons awaiting gender reassignment surgery.
- Marriage and civil partnership – the absence or presence of marriage/civil partnership can affect a person's financial and social status, and their sense of emotional well-being.
- Pregnancy and maternity – social factors can affect maternal health and perinatal outcomes as well as infant mortality.
- Race – people of different races can be more likely to encounter certain medical conditions, such as sickle cell anaemia or diabetes.
- Religion or faith – people who follow a specific diet may struggle to access specific suppliers according to their social environment. They may require prayer breaks at work and follow religious rites of passage which affect employability.
- Sex – different genders may experience different BPS needs. A female may struggle from menopausal symptoms, whilst a male is at higher risk of heart disease and has a shorter life expectancy.
- Sexual orientation – people who identify as LGBTQ + may face social prejudice and isolation and are more likely to experience poor mental health.

A programme of educational resources on personalised care and population health can be found at: www.gov.uk/government/collections/all-our-health-personalised-care-and-population-health.

Social prescribing

Social prescribing was a key component of NHS England's 'Comprehensive Model for Personalised Care' (NHSE, 2019). Within primary care, social prescribing is being used to manage long-term conditions using the BPS model. Social prescribing comes in number of different forms from walking groups, knitting meetings to support groups. Benefits of social prescribing include:

- Enabling a social connection for those that may be experiencing loneliness;
- Providing physical benefits;
- Tackling social vulnerability;
- Educational opportunities including peer support;
- Emotional well-being;
- Creating communities;
- Challenging health inequalities;
- Improving mental health;
- Reducing pressure on the NHS.

Case study 3.2: Joan part 2

Joan is becoming increasingly lonely; she has lost her appetite as it is just not appealing to eat on her own. She is socially isolated and spends long period sat in her armchair, her daughter rings a couple times a week, but she is very busy. Joan has not been able to collect her prescription so is not taking her medication. Some days she does not get dressed or eat more than a couple of rich tea biscuits; she feels like she wants to die. Her skin is beginning to feel sore on her bottom.

From the description the following physical nursing needs can be identified.

- Joan is malnourished. Action – MUST assessment, referral to dietician, dietary supplements.
- Joan is not taking her medications for pain, hypertension, and type 2 diabetes. Action – organise delivery of medications.
- Joan is not mobilising regularly, placing her at risk of pressure damage and disuse atrophy. Action – complete a pressure damage risk assessment, provide pressure relieving equipment, barrier creams, and encourage exercise.

When completing nursing care, it is important that the nursing associate also considers Joan's psycho-social needs. Patients may have different priorities in regard to their overall health and well-being. Nursing associates should ask patients what is important to them.

Case study 3.3: Joan part 3

Joan explains that she would like to be able to visit her husband's grave on their wedding anniversary. Joan's ability to achieve this goal relies on her being nutritionally stable, having controlled pain and being able to mobilise safely. Joan's GP surgery arranges for her prescription to be delivered. Joan is referred to the social prescribing team in her GP practice. Sue a local befriender begins to visit Joan. Joan enjoys the company with a cup of tea. After a few weeks Joan asks her daughter to add some 'treats' to her shopping list for when Sue visits. Joan begins to get dressed. Over time, Joan feels more confident in her mobility and Sue takes her shopping for her groceries. Joan begins to eat better; she gets stronger and feels able to socialise. She is able to visit her husband's grave.

Although social prescribing was not a traditional medical intervention, it did create positive bio-psycho-social outcomes for Joan. A model created by Moody (2009) (see Figures 3.2 and 3.3) depicts this well.

Integrated assessment

Domain	Areas to consider
Social environment	• Main carer & carer network • Next of kin & wider family • Friends & community • Preferred methods of interaction
Physical environment	• Think from the skin outwards • Clothing & footwear • Main daily living areas • Beyond the doorstep & transport
Systems of care	• Health & social care integration • Sharing information & care records • Respite & carer support • Funding & benefits
Psychological status	• Recognised conditions or symptoms • Motivation & confidence • Emotional wellbeing • Spiritual & cultural fulfilment
Multimorbidity	• Treatment burden of multiple long term conditions • Physical & mental health • Vision, hearing, dentition, continence • Strength & mobility
Acute health events	• Frailty syndromes: delirium, falls, immobility, incontinence, medication side-effects • Planned acute care (e.g. surgery)

Figure 3.2 The frailty fulcrum model

The frailty fulcrum model identifies several factors within a person's life:

- Social environment
- Physical environment
- Psychological status
- Multimorbidity (long-term conditions)
- Acute health events
- Systems of care

The model places these factors upon a scale ranging from Resilience to Vulnerability (see Figure 3.3). A person's long-term condition cannot be reversed and is likely to be placed on the vulnerability side of the scale. If other factors are not considered it is likely that they will slide down towards vulnerability too.

However, the model demonstrates how by moving some of the other factors towards the resilience end of the scale the scales may be able to balance and in turn improve a person's overall quality of life.

This model may be used by nursing associates to 'demonstrate an understanding of co-morbidities and the demands of meeting people's holistic needs when prioritising care' (NMC, 2018).

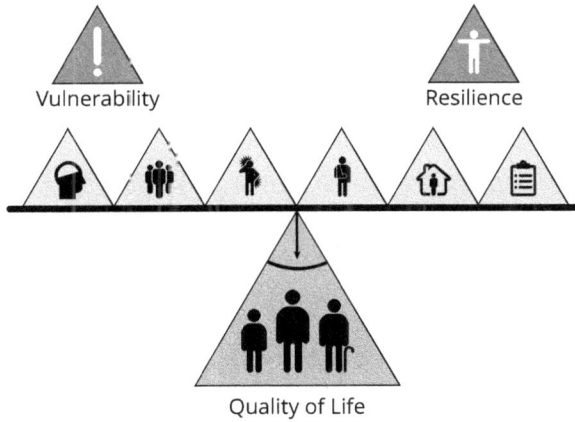

Figure 3.3   Factors that impact a person's quality of life

The role of the nursing associate in providing bio-psycho-social care

Nursing associates are well placed to provide bio-psycho-social care. The inclusion of the four domains of nursing within the qualification aids the application of the BPS model.

As we have established, a person's needs are rarely confined to only biological, psychological, or social. Healthcare professionals working in different settings need to be able to provide care for all patients. For example, people who have a learning disability will access the same healthcare settings as someone without a learning disability and therefore staff need to have the knowledge, skills, and behaviours to provide high-quality patient-centred care.

By meeting the standards of proficiency for Nursing Associates (NMC, 2018) and completing practice experience in all domains and in a range of settings, nursing associates can use their transferable knowledge accordingly.

A Nursing Associate needs to be able to utilise a range of communication tools to ensure bio-psycho-social care and to promote a person's autonomy. Example may include;

- A 'This is me' document which informs the reader of information that a person with dementia may not be able to communicate. This may include culture or religion, routines, family relations, or even how they like their tea.
- 'My Healthcare Passport'. This document provides healthcare professionals with information about a person's learning disability, how they communicate, routines, medications, allergies, long-term conditions, and anybody who should be involved in care planning.
- An advanced care plan. An advanced care plan is a document that a person has completed in anticipation of a time when they are unable to make decisions for themselves. The plan sets out their treatment preferences such as if they wish to receive cardio-pulmonary resuscitation or intravenous anti-biotics.

Separate disciplines

The separation of mental health, child, learning disability, and adult nursing disciplines within the training of nurses and in the delivery of care has arguably reinforced the belief that these are separate components of a person's health and well-being. Nursing associates are trained to work in all four disciplines and as such are well placed to bridge the gap between disciplines by utilising the BPS model. Student nursing associates (SNAs) regularly report how they can utilise transferable skills from different placement areas back to their base placement as well as sharing their experience with staff whilst on placement.

Child

Nursing associates must 'understand the importance of early years and childhood experiences and the possible impact on life choices, mental, physical and behavioural health and well-being' (NMC, 2018).

The social-cultural environment that a child lives within directly impacts upon their health. There are significant differences between children from different social economic backgrounds.

Children from a higher social economic background are more likely to play sports, eat a balanced and varied diet and be exposed to cultural experiences. Whilst children from a lower social economic background are more likely to live in a cold and damp home, eat cheap nutritionally poor foods, suffer from illness, and have poor mental health (RCPCH, 2024).

The children's health of today is the adult's health of the future. Childhood trauma and sustained levels of stress are linked to symptoms such as poor cognitive development and mental health challenges such as depression and addiction. Whilst Adverse Childhood Experiences (ACEs) have been found to directly correlate with the presence of the disease process in adulthood (Felitti, 2002), with the more ACEs experienced the higher the risk of diseases such as cancer, auto-immune conditions, and cardiac disease.

In 2018, The World Health Organization, UNICEF and The World Bank collaboratively produced the Nurturing Care Framework which identifies the components required to aid childhood development:

- The promotion of health
- A stable, safe environment
- Optimal nutrition.
- Protection from threats
- Opportunity for learning
- Affection.

These continue to be as fundamental as a child develops through adolescence with one in seven children aged 10–19 globally experiencing a mental health disorder (WHO, 2024). During adolescence children experience not only physical and emotional changes they also begin to experience different social pressures such as social inclusion, social stigma, discrimination, gender identity, and are more likely to partake in risk-taking behaviours.

Mental health

Nursing associates are required to 'demonstrate an understanding of co-morbidities and the demands of meeting people's holistic needs when prioritising care' (NMC, 2018). They are encouraged to take a person-centred approach and recognise the impact BPS needs have upon one another.

Engel's (1977) BPS model reasoned that mind and body are so intertwined that they cannot be differentiated in matters of health. Poor mental health increases the risk of long-term conditions such as cardiovascular disease, stroke and Irritable Bowel Syndrome. Similarly, the presence of a long-term condition can increase a person's risk of experiencing poor mental health. For example, a patient who has Chronic Pulmonary Obstructive Disease (COPD) is three times more likely to experience depression. This can be attributed several factors such as:

- Anxiety around being able to breathe;
- Fears surrounding death and their mortality;
- An increase in dependency;
- A change in perception of oneself.

As a nursing associate when caring for a patient with mental health needs it is important to recognise the potential side effects of medications and how they may affect the person. Some common medications used in mental health are listed below some potential side effects have been identified (not exhaustive).

Activity 3.3   Reflection

Consider how the side effects in Table 3.2 may affect a person's BPS needs.

This activity does not have a model answer.

Table 3.2   Drugs and potential side effects (BNF, 2024)

Drug	Potential side effects
Lithium	Thyroid disorders
	Mild cognitive and memory impairment
Mirtazapine	Increased appetite, joint pain, confusion, and changes to bowel habits
Sodium Valproate	Abdominal pain, alopecia, anaemia, and weight gain
Olanzapine	Hyperglycaemia, hypotension parkinsonisms, and weight gain

Learning disability

There are approximately 1.3 million people in England with a learning disability (LD) (Public Health England, 2023). People with learning disabilities have the same right to have their biological, psychological and social needs met than any other person. However, people with learning disabilities are more likely to:

- Have poorer physical health. And more likely to die up to 20 years earlier than a person without a LD. Forty-two per cent of deaths of people with a learning disability were avoidable (LeDeR, 2023);
- Have poorer mental health. Forty per cent of all people with a LD are said to have a mental health condition (NICE, 2016);
- Be living in poverty;
- Experience discrimination.

Learning Disability (LD) Nurses are registered with the NMC as their own speciality. The role has been recognised for over 100 years. LD nurses work with individuals who have a learning disability to meet their BPS needs. However, the Royal College of Nursing (RCN, 2024) have revealed that the number of LD nurses has fallen from 5,553 some 15 years ago to 3,095 in 2024. The reduction in LD nurses leaves a deficit in provision.

All areas and specialities within the health service provide care for people with learning disabilities. Therefore, it is imperative that all nursing associates have experience of learning disability nursing and recognise the most significant factors to be conscious of when providing, monitoring and delivering care (NMC, 2023) whilst also recognising the person as an individual.

Activity 3.4   Reflection

Consider your place of work. What adaptations do you have in place for a people with a learning disability?

- Do you have easy read patient information?
- How can appointments be accessed?
- How may you introduce the environment?
- What sensory considerations are there?

As this activity is based on your own observation, there is no outline answer at the end of the chapter.

Nursing associates need to be able to recognise and accommodate sensory impairments. Every person with autism is an individual and presumptions should not be made due to a diagnosis. However, it is important to be aware of sensory considerations.

- People with autism can have an altered responsivity to pain. They can be hyposensitive or hypersensitive to pain.
- Children with autism can have a heightened sense of smell.
- People with autism can have a taste sensitivity. They may only like a particular brand or type of food and can recognise when there is a difference. They may struggle to take oral medications.
- Some sounds can be particularly overwhelming for people with autism. The call bells on a ward, the sounds of machines and the telephone ringing can all add to a person with autism's discomfort.
- Some textures maybe uncomfortable for a person with autism, this may be the bedding or hospital gown for example.
- Some people with autism have an avoidance to touch – examinations, observations, and clinical investigations may be difficult for a person with autism.

Public Health England (2023) provide guidance on communicating with people with a learning difficulty to promote their autonomy and health literacy. Please note that this is supportive guidance and does not replace a patient centered approach. Nursing Associates need to be able to adapt their communication style to meet the needs of the individual.

- Always speak directly to the person, unless advised not to do so.
- Use plain English, short sentences and do not use medical jargon and acronyms.
- Ask if they have a hospital passport – this may include information on their preferred method of communicating with others.
- Use visual aids such as photographs, objects, or gestures to support your words, and make use of supplementary NHS YouTube videos.

- Ask if they use any alternative forms of communication, such as Makaton (signs and speech), Talking Mats (symbols), Beyond Words (wordless picture books) or symbol-based images, like Widgit – if you are not able to use their tools, ask if they have someone with them who can assist.
- When writing, make it accessible to the individual – this may mean using larger, easy-to-read text to explain what you wish to say and easy read appointment letters (the NIHR website has advice on accessible health information).
- Talk and listen to the person's carer, friend or supporting professional, without excluding the individual.
- Give the person time (ideally seven seconds) to process what you have said before they respond.
- Check understanding, both yours and the person's, by asking open questions.
- Pay attention to body language and facial expressions.
- Consider the environment – noisy or loud environments with lots of activity are not conducive to effective communication.
- Show any equipment or machines that might be used and explain any noise that the machines may make to pre-empt any problems.
- Offer to follow up verbal discussions with a written note or a voice or video recording.

Case study 3.2: Ben

Ben is 12 and has autism, tonight is a Thursday, and he normally watches Darts. However, he has been admitted to hospital because of acute abdominal pain. He is in a side room and his mum is staying with him. However, Ben is becoming increasingly anxious. Ben is holding his ears and rocking back and forth.

It is important to note that every person with autism is an individual and presumptions should not be made due to a diagnosis. However, the examples below aim to highlight some sensory considerations that maybe experienced by a person who has Autism in an inpatient setting.

People with Autism could have a heightened sense of smell.

Activity 3.5 Discussion

Discuss potential bio-psycho-social factors that may be affecting Ben. Consider how you could use a person-centred approach when delivering Ben's care.

This activity does not have a model answer.

The spiritual model

A limitation of the bio-psycho-social model is the absence of a recognition of a person's spiritual needs. Holistic care involves caring for a person's overall wellbeing including their spirituality. There are a range of definitions of what is spirituality. This is because spirituality means different things to different people. Some people may link the concept of spirituality to their religion or faith whilst others may use it to describe a connection to something cosmic or divine in nature. Spirituality is linked to personal growth and wellbeing and may be demonstrated through pray, mindfulness or a connection with nature. Some individuals will not describe themselves as spiritual and may instead refer to themselves as an Atheist or Agnostic; nevertheless, a holistic approach to overall wellbeing is required.

Due to the diversity in the spiritual needs of individuals, as nursing associates it is important to be able to *Reflect on people's values and beliefs, diverse backgrounds, cultural characteristics, language requirements, needs and preferences, taking account of any need for adjustments'* (NMC, 2018).

Patients are likely to rely on their spirituality to help them cope with periods of ill health or when needing to adapt to significant life changes. The concept of spiritual care within nursing practice has been attributed to Battey (2009). However, history illustrates how nursing has always been linked to spiritual and religious care with the nursing role frequently being referred as a 'calling'.

Understanding the theory

The Spiritual Nursing Care Theory Model created by Bangcola (2021) depicts how a person's spirituality is integral to holism and just as essential as any other need. The theoretical framework is composed of four components:

1. Spiritual nursing care
2. The nurse's spiritual competency
3. The cultural background of the patient
4. The patient's spiritual needs.

Within clinical practice, nursing associates need to be able to provide care that recognises a person's spirituality. A healthcare professional is not expected to know all cultural, religious, values and beliefs but they are expected to utilise effective communication with the person to find out their needs. When a person is unable to communicate their spiritual needs, healthcare professionals should liaise with their families. There may be differences within different cultures or religions, so it is always better to ask, rather than presume what a person needs.

The HOPE assessment tool was established by Anandarajah and Hight in 2001.
HOPE stands for.

H- Hope. What are your sources of hope, strength, and comfort? Thinking back to the challenging times in your life, what or who has helped you cope and get through these times?

O- Organised Religion. Are you part of a spiritual or religious community? If so, does being part of this community help you? In what ways? Does it help you? How? What spiritual practices or beliefs help you?

P- Personal spiritual practice. (Prayer, Meditation, Scripture, Worship, Music, Art, Nature, etc.) How do you feel you're doing spiritually? How is it with your soul?

E- Effects on your Care. As your nurse, what can I do to help honour your spiritual/religious needs? As you face this challenge in your life, how can your religious community, (or health care team or other resources) help honour your spiritual/religious needs?

Other spiritual considerations include.

- Dietary needs;
- The gender of the healthcare professional providing care;
- The availability of space for pray and/or meditation;
- Washing facilities;
- The use of eye contact;
- Language;
- The role of family members;
- Last rites;
- Clothes and personal presentation.

Chapter summary

Providing person-centred care which encompasses a person's bio-psycho-social and spiritual needs is a rewarding experience. Building a therapeutic relationship with patients and their families enables you to meet their individual holistic needs and encompasses overall health and wellbeing. Going forward you are encouraged to replace 'what is the matter with you?' with 'what matters to you?'

'the good physician treats the disease; the great physician treats the patient who has the disease'

William Osler, 1849–1919.

Chapter 4

Understanding assessment tools

Hazel Cowls

Chapter aims

After reading this chapter you will be able to:

- Discuss the purpose of assessment tools;
- Understand terms associated with assessment tools such as reliability, validity, specificity, and sensitivity;
- Explain the importance of using assessment tools in clinical practice when assessing a person's needs.

Introduction

In Chapter 3, you looked at the theory and principles of the bio-psycho-social model and understood how this model supports a person-centred approach. As a student nursing associate (SNA) or registered nursing associate (RNA), you may be familiar with a range of assessment tools that will enable you to deliver direct care, with minimal supervision, using your knowledge and skills to make effective clinical decisions (NMC, 2024). For example, the assessment tools that you have seen in practice will provide you with a baseline assessment of a person's nutritional state, hydration, skin integrity, falls prevention risk assessment, wound assessments, and many more. These assessment tools will aid your clinical assessment and decision-making, informing you of an appropriate plan of action and care. In this chapter, you will explore the purpose of assessment tools, understand the validity and specificity of different tools used in a variety of clinical settings and fields of nursing associate practice.

The purpose of an assessment tool

Assessment tools are simply a series of questions to the people receiving care, family members and health and social care professionals. The answers to these questions may be a rating scale, a yes or no, or specific measures of concern that are intended to provide an estimate of the severity of concern (Ellis et al., 2020). Assessment tools help us to gather specific clinical data to aid a clinical decision that will determine the need for patient interventions or actions and whether interventions have been successful. Sometimes the evaluation may show that the intervention is not working, and there may be a need to consider an alternative intervention. By obtaining this information the health and social care team can ascertain a balanced patient assessment that will lead to a person-centred and robust plan of care. This will be discussed in more detail in Chapter 6 when we look at the principles and theories of planning nursing care.

Assessment tools can be used for health screening, to aid a diagnosis, or to predict ill health (screening, diagnostic or predictive). Assessment tools enable us to gather a lot of information quickly. There are many names given to assessment tools such as:

- Clinical assessment tools
- Screening tools or screening instruments
- Risk assessment tools
- Clinical algorithms

Screening tools or screening instruments – is there a difference?

A dictionary definition of a tool 'is any instrument or device necessary to one's profession or occupation' (Collins English Dictionary n.d.). Essentially, a screening tool or instrument are the same. Health screening is essential in preventative medicine; screening tools or instruments will identify people early who may be at risk of developing a condition. Health screening aids early identification to provide treatment and reduce any symptoms, therefore improving health outcomes (Iragorri and Spackman, 2018). A lot of health screening can be carried out effectively in general practice such as electrocardiography, blood pressure and blood tests. Effective health screening is also cost effective; if illness is identified early enough and symptoms are treated early, then this may be less expensive for health organisations. In fact, many countries have developed national screening programmes, such as breast screening in the United Kingdom (Blanks et al., 1998). The benefits of health screening and national screening programmes are to detect a problem early, sometimes even before symptoms have developed. Health screening can reduce the chance of developing a condition or complications, and prevent death from abdominal aortic aneurysms, breast cancer, bowel cancer, and cervical cancer. For the public, health screening enables them to make informed decisions about their health and the treatment options (National Health Service [NHS], 2021). The UK National Screening Committee (UK NSC), an independent expert group, advises ministers and the National Health Service in the four UK countries on which screening programmes to offer. Table 4.1 shows examples of health screening programmes carried out in the United Kingdom.

Table 4.1   Health screening in the United Kingdom

Screening programmes	
Screening in pregnancy	For infectious diseases
	For Down's syndrome
	To check the development of the baby
	Diabetic eye screening if you have type 1 or 2 diabetes
	Assessment and diagnosis of a suspected mental health problem in pregnancy and the postnatal period
For babies	Newborn blood spot (NBS) screening programme
	Newborn and infant physical examination (NIPE) screening programme
	Newborn hearing screening programme (NHSP)
	Sickle cell and thalassaemia (SCT) screening programme
For children	Vision tests, your child's eyes may be checked several times throughout the first hours, weeks and years of their life.
	Children may also have a hearing test as part of their development checks.
Diabetic eye screening	From the age of 12, people with diabetes are offered annual diabetic eye screening to check for retinopathy
Cervical screening	Offered to all women and people with a cervix aged 25–64 to check the health of cells in the cervix (aged 25–59 every three years; 50–64 every five years)
Breast screening	Offered to women aged 50–71 to detect early signs of breast cancer every three years. If you're a trans man, trans woman or are non-binary you may be invited automatically, or you may need to talk to your GP surgery or call the local breast screening service to ask for an appointment. Over 71 years and you can request screening.
Bowel cancer screening	Home screening kit offered to people 54–74 every two years

However, the risks and limitations of screening are that it is not 100 per cent accurate. For example, someone could be told that they have a problem, when they do not, and this is known as a *false positive*. In contrast, a person could be told that they do not have a problem when in fact they do, and this is known as a *false negative*. Many false positives and negatives may lead to the need for other diagnostic tests and delays in a confirmed diagnosis (see Figure 4.1).

	Disease positive	Disease negative
Positive test (screening)	True positive	False positive
Negative test	False negative	True negative

Figure 4.1   Understanding the sensitivity and specificity of tests

Understanding the sensitivity and specificity of tests will be discussed in more detail later in this chapter but it is worth remembering that depending upon the tests results a person may need to undergo additional predictive or diagnostic tests and, depending on the nature of the test, these may not be risk free. For example, a person needs to have medical imaging that uses radioactive dye (known as a tracer), and although radioactive dye is generally safe, some people may experience adverse side effects such as headache, nausea, flushing, hypersensitivity, or rash (Joint Formulary Committee, 2025).

Activity 4.1   Critical thinking

Choose one example of health screening carried out in the United Kingdom. What patient information is available about this test? Is the patient information clear?

There is no outline answer at the end of the chapter.

As a SNA and RNA, it is useful to know which screening programmes are relevant to your area of practice. Being able to understand the process of referral to screening, as well as the specifics of any tests, are essential if you are directly involved in a screening programme as you can support people who are waiting for screening tests. Unfortunately, not everyone has access to health screening (health inequalities) due to location, or a lack of knowledge about the screening programme. Therefore, you may be able to educate people about the benefits of health screening that could increase people's adherence, leading to early identification of disease and treatment. Health inequalities is an important topic and will be discussed in more detail in Chapter 7.

The case study below illustrates how a SNA can work with service users as well as other healthcare professionals to ensure family centred care is delivered.

Case Study 4.1: Aadhya

Mum has brought Aadhya aged four months old to a paediatric outpatient clinic for her second hearing test. The clinic is run by an audiologist, a registered nurse (child) and a SNA, who is supporting the RN. The SNA notices that mum is looking apprehensive and approaches her to inquire how she is. Mum states that she is worried her baby is not developing as expected as she rarely makes any noises or gurgling sounds. She is worried that Aadhya may have permanent hearing loss. Mum asks about the test and whether her baby will be uncomfortable during the test. The SNA reassures mum that her baby will not be uncomfortable and that she can stay with Aadhya for the duration of the test. The average duration of a hearing test is up to an hour. The SNA explains that the audiologist will explain the results of the test at the end of the appointment and whether any further tests are required.

The SNA informed the RN and audiologist about mum's fears. This information will be helpful to the audiologist and RN as they will ensure that mum has time during the consultation to ask any questions.

Activity 4.2   Critical thinking

You have read the case study about Aadhya above. As a SNA, how else can you support mum and prepare Aadhya for her hearing test?

An outline answer is given at the end of this chapter.

Risk assessment tools

Risk assessment tools aim to predict whether a person may develop a problem for example, a pressure sore using a pressure risk assessment tool. The following are evidence-based pressure risk assessment tools to support clinical judgement when assessing pressure ulcer risk in adults:

- Brandon Risk Assessment
- PURPOSE-T (Pressure Ulcer Risk Primary or Secondary Evaluation Tool)
- Waterlow assessment
- Brandon Q Scale (for children) (National Institute for Health and Care Excellence [NICE], 2024)

Each risk assessment tool predicts a person's level of risk depending on a person's characteristics condition, sensory perception, mobility and medication. The risk assessment tools are interdisciplinary and will guide healthcare professionals on a specific management plan to reduce risk of pressure damage.

Understanding the theory: Risk assessment tools

Table 4.2   Risk assessment tools

Risk assessment tool	Purpose of tool
Brancon Q Scale	Suitable to use on paediatric population. Seven key components are mobility, activity, sensory perception, moisture, nutrition, tissue perfusion, and oxygen and friction.
Brandon Risk Assessment	Suitable to use on adult population and key components as listed above.
PURPOSE-T	Identifies people at risk but also those with existing or previous pressure ulcers requiring secondary prevention treatment. Three-step approach to assessing risk and treatment.
Waterlow assessment	Suitable to use on adult population. Twelve key components to the risk assessment that include gender, age, body mass index (BMI), skin type, mobility, continence, recent weight loss, poor appetite, tissue malnutrition, neurological deficit, major trauma or surgery, and medication.

Another example of a risk assessment tool is the falls risk assessment tool (FRAT) that will look at a person's age, history of falls, psychological and cognitive status, medication, and mobility. There are several clinical areas where you may need to complete a FRAT such as in an acute hospital, community hospital or in a person's home. Completion of a FRAT will identify which category a person falls into and how much support is required. Therefore, we can see how risk assessment tools enable us to provide person-centred, high-quality, safe patient care.

Clinical algorithms

A clinical algorithm is a 'process' or set of 'rules' to be followed to aid clinical decision-making and the management of a clinical problem (Margolis, 1983). The 'rules' are based on the best evidence available and are agreed at either a national or local level. A care bundle and a care pathway are examples of clinical algorithms. A care bundle is a structured way of improving care and patient outcomes using three to five evidence-based interventions. Whereas a care pathway explains the process from referral (usually by the GP) to diagnostics and care management, a care pathway will often include multi-agencies and is also agreed at a national and local level. Both examples will be discussed in more detail in Chapter 6.

Understanding the terms associated with assessment tools

All assessment tools must be reliable and valid, as when used correctly with the specific patient group, they will help the nurse in making clinical decisions about the person's care. *Reliability* is associated with the ability of an assessment tool to produce accurate and consistent results under similar circumstances (Glasper and Rees, 2017). For example, a numerical pain rating scale (NPRS) is an 11-point self-assessment pain scale (rating from 0 = no pain; 1–3 = mild pain; 4–6 = moderate pain 7–10 = severe pain). The advantages of the NPRS are it is easy to explain, score and takes a few minutes to complete. The NPRS has been shown to be reliable for the older person or people with lower literacy (Ferraz et al., 1990).

Validity refers to the ability of a healthcare assessment to measure what it intends to measure. For example, the National Early Warning Score 2 (NEWS2) is an aggregated scoring system allocated to physiological measurements that is used as a track and trigger system to assess person's level of illness and signs of deterioration. The scoring system is used in acute hospitals, emergency departments, and pre-hospitals. The validity of NEWS2 lies in the extensive research carried out by the Royal College of Physicians (2017). As a SNA/RNA recording and interpreting the physiological data you must be trained to measure each physiological parameter (oxygen saturation, blood pressure, pulse, respiratory rate, level of consciousness, and temperature) and trained to input the data onto the NEWS2 chart.

Other factors that influence the results of assessments are the intra-reliability and inter-rater reliability of the assessment tools being used to collect the data. Intra-reliability refers to the same person carrying out a re-assessment using the same tool. Whereas inter-rater reliability refers to the degree of agreement or consistency of results amongst raters or observers. For example, measuring subjective factors such as pain can be difficult to capture as people experience symptoms differently. For example, you are looking after a person post-surgical procedure and using a validated verbal rating pain assessment scale. The patient reports a pain scale rating of 5 out of 10 but how is this interpreted?

Assessment tools need to be sensitive enough to identify people that may be at risk, for example identifying a person experiencing severe acute anxiety from a sample of 100 people. But they also need to be specific enough that it does not pick up everyone, only those with severe acute anxiety. One assessment tool that is used to identify people with acute anxiety are the Generalised Anxiety Disorder 7 (GAD-7). This assessment tool will be discussed in more detail later in the chapter.

Understand the theory

A summary of the terms associated with assessment tools

Sensitivity:

- Does it correctly identify all cases?

Specificity:

- Does it correctly identify all cases?

Reliability:

- Does it provide consistent results?

Validity:

- Does it measure what it claims to measure?

Intra-reliability:

- If repeated by the same person, the result will be consistent

Inter-rater reliability:

- If repeated by the same person, the result will be consistent

The importance of using assessment tools in practice

In this section, you will recognise the importance of using assessment tools in practice by looking at specific case studies across different fields of nursing associate practice and reflecting on your own practice as a SNA.

Case Study 4.2: Adrianna

Adrianna is 10 years old and has been admitted to the Children Assessment Unit following a history of feeling sick, fever and abdominal pain. Adrianna has been seen by the admitting doctor and a prescription has been written that includes analgesia.

You are the SNA looking after Adrianna. Her mother reports that Adrianna still has abdominal pain, and she is worried about her. You assess Adrianna's level of pain using the Wong-Baker FACES Pain Rating Scale developed in 1983 (see Figure 4.2). An accurate assessment of pain is essential when managing pain as you need to establish the current pain score, administer treatment if prescribed and then re-assess to establish whether treatment has been effective.

Adrianna points to emoji number 6 on the pain scale, you inform the RN, and with the RN's supervision administer the prescribed analgesia. You advise Adrianna and her mother that it may take a short time for the analgesia to take effect and that you will return to reassess. On your return to review Adrianna's level of pain, Adrianna points to emoji number 2.

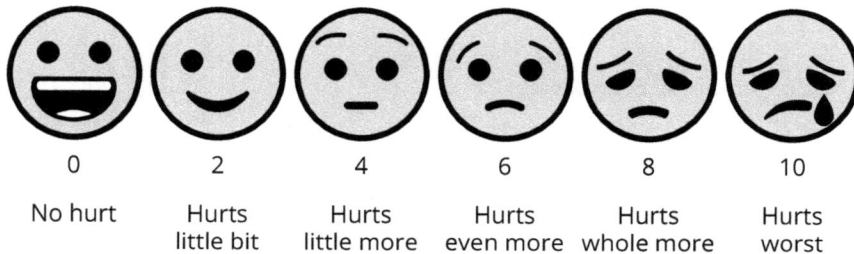

0	2	4	6	8	10
No hurt	Hurts little bit	Hurts little more	Hurts even more	Hurts whole more	Hurts worst

Figure 4.2 Wong-Baker® Faces Pain Rating Scale – www.WongBakerFACES.org

This assessment tool is an example of a visual analogue scale (VAS). Generally, a VAS is straight 100-mm line, that has the words 'no pain to worst pain imaginable' or something similar and is relatively simple to explain to the user and to interpret. In this case study, the SNA asks Adrianna to report her pain using the 'Faces' pain rating scale. The 'Faces' pain rating scale is a simple tool that can be used when assessing a child's pain (Wong and Baker, 1998) and has been shown to be both reliable and valid (Bieri et al., 1990; Garra et al., 2010).

A numerical rating scale (NRS) or numerical pain rating scale (NPRS) is another example of a pain assessment tool. The NRS is one of the simplest and most used pain assessment scales and is like a VAS. The numerical scale consists of numbers and verbal prompts across a range of possible responses (Lazaridou et al., 2018). The numbers are spaced evenly across a chart and patients are instructed to circle one of the numbers to rate their pain from 0 to 10, with 0 being 'no pain' and 10 being 'the worst pain imaginable'. The advantages of NRS pain assessment tools are that they are relatively simple, easy to understand, and children as young as five years old recognise that the number eight is larger than four (Iohom, 2006). A criticism of the NRS is that for some people it can be difficult to quantify pain between 0 to 10 as the range is too broad, some people find it easier to use a NRS of 0–3 with verbal prompts no pain; mild pain; moderate pain; and severe pain – no pain (0); mild pain (1); moderate pain (2); and severe pain (3). Some people with a motor disability may find it difficult to record their score and may need to use a verbal rating scale.

A verbal rating scale (VRS) is also like visual analogue and numerical rating scales where patients are asked to rate their pain either 0 to 10 or using verbal descriptors such as no pain to severe pain. However, numerical, verbal and visual pain assessment scales are unidimensional, and there are other more sophisticated scales that address other dimensions of pain, known as multidimensional assessment scales.

Activity 4.3   Research

There are different types of pain assessment tools – research other types of pain rating scales, or assessment tools that may be relevant to your practice. Consider the following: is the assessment tool easy to use and explain to others? Have you been shown how to use the assessment tool? Do you feel confident showing someone else how to use the assessment tool?

As this activity is based on your own observation, there is no outline answer at the end of the chapter.

Multidimensional pain assessment scales address multiple domains of pain, for example, sensory, impact, and temporal components. You may come across multidimensional pain assessment tools if you are working with a specialist pain team or clinic environment as the specialist teams will be looking at the domains of pain and how this may be impacting a person's life. Examples of multidimensional pain assessment tools include the McGill Pain Questionnaire (MPQ) and the Brief Pain Inventory (BPI). The MPQ (Melzack, 1975) provided a breakthrough in pain assessment as pain assessment was no longer seen as one-dimensional as the qualitative aspect of pain became important. The MPQ included 78 words to describe three different dimensions of pain:

1. The sensory aspect of pain in terms of temporal, spacial, and pressure
2. The affective qualities in terms of tension and fear
3. The evaluative quality of pain that described the overall intensity of pain

The shortened MPQ known as SF-MPQ (Shortened Form -McGill Pain Questionnaire) (Melzack, 1987) consists of two domains (sensory and affective) and 15-word descriptors (11 sensory; 4 affective) that are rated on an intensity scale of 0–3. The SF-MPQ has been shown to be a useful tool when the standard MPQ takes too long to administer, yet qualitative information is desired, and a VAS is seen as inadequate (Melzack, 1987).

The Brief Pain Inventory (BPI) is available in either a long (17 items) or short (nine items) form. The BPI focuses on pain severity and pain interference, that is how does pain interfere with a person's feelings and function. The shortened form (BPI-sf) is a self-administered questionnaire, and the patient is asked to record their pain intensity, their treatment and perceived effectiveness, and the impact the pain has on their functioning such as work, play and sleep. Initially, the BPI form was intended for people experiencing cancer related pain but is now used for people with non-malignant pain such as post-surgery, osteoarthritis, and neuropathy.

Activity 4.4   Research

Read about the McGill Pain Questionnaire or Brief Pain Inventory or another multidimensional assessment tool that is relevant to your area of practice.

As this activity is based on your own observation, there is no outline answer at the end of the chapter.

> ## Case Study 4.3: Meena
>
> You are a SNA and attend a home visit with the Health Visitor to see Meena and her baby, Caleb, who is now nine weeks old. Meena's two-year-old daughter is also present. The planned visit is the mandatory 6–8 week visit and aims to focus on the baby's growth and the health of the parents. Baby Caleb looks well and is meeting weight expectations. Meena is responding appropriately and warmly to Caleb's needs. However, you notice Meena looks visibly tired, she is wearing dishevelled clothing that is too big for her, and her general appearance and body odour suggest that she may not have addressed her self-care needs. Meena discloses that she is forgetting things, even eating, and feels useless. She admits to leaving Caleb in his cot, so she can get a rest, and she talks about struggling to manage both children, saying 'I dread being left alone with them and I dread going out with them'. Meena reports that she is worried other people will think she isn't taking good enough care of her children. Meena is struggling to feel positive about the future. She describes extremely poor sleep due to having two children night waking. Meena denies any perceptual disturbances, intrusive thoughts, or suicidal ideation.

Assessing a woman for depression during pregnancy and during the postnatal period is essential for the early detection and appropriate management. Some points to consider are:

1. Is there a history of anxiety or depression?
2. What social support is available?
3. Are there any other factors such as illness that may impact on a person's mental health?

In Meena's case, there are a few indicators that she may be feeling anxious or depressed. She reports sleep disturbances, worrying, not eating, and you have observed that she may not be looking after her own self-care needs. The first step in an assessment such as this, is to establish whether mum is at risk of harm to self and others. Meena does not report any perceptual disturbances (hallucinations or disorganised thinking) and there is no risk of harm to baby, Meena denies any suicidal ideation. The next step is to establish the severity of possible depression to establish whether further intervention is required. The Edinburgh Postnatal Depression Scale (EPDS) (Cox et al., 1987) is a validated tool to assess postpartum (postnatal) depression. The EPDS was developed to aid healthcare professionals in detecting whether a mother was experiencing symptoms of postnatal depression and is used internationally. The scale is relatively simple to explain and is self-administered, taking several minutes to complete. The scale consists of ten short statements and a mother would tick the response that she is currently experiencing. The EPDS responses are scored from 0 to 3 based on the seriousness, maximum aggregated score is 30, and a score greater than 12 or 13 suggests that the mother may be suffering with depression (Cox et al., 1987). The scale indicates how the mother felt the previous week, so it may be necessary to repeat the scale. The EPDS is not a diagnostic tool and therefore the mother would need to be reviewed by a relevant healthcare professional to confirm a diagnosis and establish a treatment plan. An example of the type of questions used in this questionnaire would be 'I have been able to laugh and see the funny side of things':

- As much as I always could
- Not quite as much now
- Definitely not so much now
- Not at all

Another assessment tool that is used in mental health and a variety of clinical settings is the Generalised Anxiety Disorder (GAD-7), a self-administered questionnaire that asks people to complete how they have been feeling over the last two weeks and due to the simple language used this tool can be used from 14 years upwards (Spitzer et al., 2006). The GAD-7 is a screening tool to measure level of anxiety and consists of seven statements and a total score is calculated by assigning a score of 0–3 to the responses. The questions relate to whether a person has been feeling anxious, nervous, worrying, has trouble relaxing or feeling restless and the frequency of these emotions. The responses to each of the questions are:

- Not at all
- Several days
- More than half the days
- Nearly every day

The GAD-7 is normally used in a primary care setting or in an outpatient department either face to face or during a virtual or telephone consultation. The results of a GAD-7 may indicate mild, moderate or severe anxiety and is moderately good at screening other common anxiety disorders such as panic disorder (sensitivity 74 per cent, specificity 81 per cent); post-traumatic stress disorder (sensitivity 66 per cent, specificity 81 per cent) and social anxiety disorder (sensitivity 72 per cent, specificity 80 per cent) (Kroenke et al., 2007). The assessment tool can identify people who may need to be referred to a service, or for a person who is receiving treatment, the results will be part of an evaluation (is the treatment having a positive effect on a person's well-being). The anxiety scores using GAD-7 are as follows:

- 0–4 (no anxiety)
- 5–9 (mild anxiety)
- 10–14 (moderate anxiety)
- 15–21 (severe anxiety)

Another assessment tool used to monitor the severity of depressive symptoms is the Patient Healthcare Questionnaire (PHQ-9), (Kroenke et al., 2001). The PHQ-9 is a self-administered patient questionnaire and asks people to record how they have been feeling over the last two weeks. The questions relate to a how a person feels about themselves, their sleep pattern, their energy levels and eating habits. The responses to each of the questions are:

- Not at all
- Several days
- More than half the days
- Nearly every day

The validity of PHQ-9 has been assessed against an interview conducted by an independent mental health professional and the PHQ-9 score $\geq$10 (moderate depression) had 88 per cent sensitivity and 88 per cent specificity for depression (Kroenke et al., 2001). Not only can this questionnaire be self-administered in a clinic setting or primary care but also over the telephone (Pinto-Meza et al., 2005). Being able to confidently assess a person's mental well-being over the telephone ensures that healthcare assessment is available to all, whether this is due to immobility, inaccessibility, physical or mental health illness. During the SARS-CoV-2 pandemic the practice of completing assessments over the telephone would have increased compared to previous years. The depression severity scores using anxiety scores using PHQ-9 are as follows:

- 0–4 (no depression)
- 5–9 (mild depression)
- 10–14 (moderate depression)
- 15–19 (moderately severe depression)
- 20–27 (severe depression)

As a SNA or RNA, you may ask a person to complete a GAD-7 questionnaire or PHQ-9, and you may need to explain the rationale for completing the form whether it is pre-treatment or part of ongoing management.

Finally, a Mental State Examination (MSE), not to be confused with a *mini-mental state examination* (MMSE) which is a 30-point cognitive screening tool used in clinical and research settings (please see further reading on MMSE). The MSE is not really an 'assessment tool' but rather an approach to completing a holistic assessment providing a structured framework for assessing a person's mental well-being. If you are carrying out a mental state examination, you will be observing how a person appears, their behaviour, speech, mood, movement, expression of thought, perception, and cognition. Take a moment to reflect on a time when you saw a patient or client, what did you notice first about the person? For example, you are visiting a person in their own home, what do you notice? Alternatively, you are seeing a person in a clinic setting, how do they walk into your clinic room, are they able to explain their symptoms clearly to you, do they understand you? Do they appear angry or cross? Finally, you may see a person in a community or acute hospital setting, do you notice any signs of alcohol or substance misuse? Have you noticed any abnormal movement or postures? What is the person's body language telling you? Are you aware of any abnormalities of perception?

Activity 4.5   Research

Have a look at the mental state examination and make some notes on key observations. Consider what questions you would ask someone.

An outline answer is given at the end of this chapter.

Registered nursing associate voice 4.1

When speaking with a RNA about the benefits of assessment tools in practice, they stated that:

Assessment tools provide a universal way of assessment. We cannot practise effectively and safely without them.

Activity 4.6   Critical thinking

Find one or two assessment tools that are used in your clinical area. Research the assessment tool and answer the following questions. How was the tool developed? What is the assessment tool measuring? Is this assessment tool: a) a screening tool, b) a diagnostic tool, c) a predictive tool? As a SNA, do you feel confident using the assessment tool?

There is no outline answer at the end of the chapter.

What are the benefits and limitations of assessment tools?

The benefits of all assessment tools are that they provide quantifiable clinical data as opposed to an opinion. The clinical data can be obtained in a short space of time, to enable clinicians to act quickly if needed and this in turn will improve patient care. The data can also allow a comparison between the person receiving care and the norms of the populations (specific or general population). For example, a person's blood pressure recorded at 120/80 mm Hg (millimetres of mercury) is considered within the normal range. The data can also be viewed over time and can also be interpreted at a later stage. For example, you may be asked to check a person's blood pressure whilst in hospital or if they are attending a GP surgery as they are known to have hypertension (high blood pressure) and have recently started anti-hypertensive medication.

As a SNA and RNA, you need to understand the purpose of the assessment tool; what is the tool assessing, is the information objective or subjective, how is the assessment tool completed and interpreted. Any inaccuracies in completing assessment tools may lead to errors in treatment, for example. You also need to be aware of your own clinical judgement; for example, a person could be experiencing significant abdominal pain and feeling dizzy but remain normotensive (normal blood pressure) when lying down. However, when the person tries to stand up there may be a drop in blood pressure (orthostatic hypotension); this, associated with abdominal pain, may indicate internal bleeding depending on other clinical signs and history. Clinical judgement and clinical decision-making will be discussed in more detail in Chapter 5.

Activity 4.7   Reflection

Using Gibbs' model of reflection, describe a time when you have used an assessment tool. The steps of Gibbs' model of reflection are:

1. Describe the situation
2. How did you feel?

(Continued)

3. What was good and bad about the situation?
4. What sense can you make of the situation?
5. What have you learnt and what could you do better?
6. What is your action plan?

Remember to include whether the assessment tool is: a) a screening tool, b) a diagnostic tool, c) a predictive tool.

As this activity is based on your own observation, there is no outline answer at the end of the chapter.

Registered nurse associate voice 4.2

When discussing the limitations of assessment tools, the RNA mentioned that assessment tools may not show the whole picture.

Remember an assessment tool is a guide, the data may be normal, but you may be worried about your patient. Go with that feeling, that is your clinical judgement.

Chapter summary

This chapter has explored the purpose of assessment tools for health screening, predictive or diagnostics, across different fields of practice. Assessment tools are generally a series of questions that can be answered by the patient, family member, parent or carer. Assessment tools enable you to gather a lot of patient information quickly and can provide a general estimate for severity or concern. There are three main reasons we use assessment tools: a) screening, b) predictive, c) diagnostic. The case studies have provided additional information to help contextualise the use of assessment tools in your practice as a SNA/RNA. The activities have provided you with an opportunity to become familiar with assessment tools used in your own practice and to develop a deeper understanding of the tools that are used not only in your own practice but elsewhere.

Activities: Brief outline answers

Activity 4.2 Critical thinking (page 59)

You may have considered communication skills and building rapport with Mum so that she feels comfortable speaking with you. You could explain that there are two types of hearing tests that are otoacoustic emissions test (OAE) and auditory brainstem response (ABR). The OAE test is carried out by placing a small earpiece, containing a speaker and a microphone, in Aadhya's ear. A clicking sound is played and if the cochlea is working properly the microphone in the earpiece will pick up the response. The test is recorded on a computer and informs the audiologist whether a response is present or not. If Aadhya has a clear response during her hearing test, then she will not need any more tests. A poor response to a hearing test does not necessarily mean that a child is deaf. Other factors such as the baby being unsettled at the time of the test, a noisy room or fluid in the baby's ear may lead to a poor test result. You could recommend that Mum feed baby before or change her nappy so that she is settled before the test. As the SNA, you could also suggest Mum thinks about her questions to ask the audiologist.

The ABR measures whether sound is being sent from the cochlea (inner ear) and through the auditory (hearing) nerve to the brain.

Activity 4.5 Research (page 66)

A mental state examination will consider a person's appearance, their behaviour, speech, mood, thoughts, perception, insights and judgement, and risk to themselves. An example of what you may have considered:

Observation	What do you notice?	What could you ask?
Appearance	Evidence of neglect.	Substance misuse: what do they use?
	Signs of alcohol or substance use.	Self-neglect: are they eating and drinking?
		Are they attending to their physical health needs? (e.g., taking medications for physical health conditions)
Cognition	Is the person orientated in time, place and person?	What year is it?
		What is your date of birth?
	What their attention span and concentration levels are like?	Do you know where you are?
	What their short-term memory is like?	Who is the prime minister?
Insight and Judgement	Person may appear distracted or focussing on something particular	What do you think the cause of the problem is?
		Do you think you have a problem now?
		Do you feel you need help with your problem?

Useful websites

BAPEN. Introducing Malnutrition Universal Screening Tool' (MUST). Available at: www.bapen.org.uk/must-and-self-screening/introducing-must/

A valuable resource for learning about the 'Malnutrition Universal Screening Tool' (MUST), how to identify people who may be at nutritional risk or potentially at risk, and who may benefit from appropriate nutritional intervention.

National Institute for Healthcare Excellence Clinical Guideline 179, Pressure ulcers: prevention and management. Available at: www.nice.org.uk/guidance/cg179/resources

Tools and resources to enable you to apply the guidance to your clinical practice. Includes links to algorithms for risk management, prevention and management in adults and children.

NHS Screening. Available at: www.nhs.uk/conditions/nhs-screening/

This page gives an overview of health screening and links to screening offered to people within the NHS in England.

NHS Mental Health Assessments. Available at: www.nhs.uk/mental-health/social-care-and-your-rights/mental-health-assessments/

This page gives an overview of mental health assessments and includes a link to the Mental Health Act.

Royal College of Physicians - NEWS2. Available at: www.rcplondon.ac.uk/projects/outputs/national-early-warning-score-news-2

Information on NEWS2, the aggregate scoring system in which a score is allocated to physiological measurements, when patients present to, or are being monitored in hospital. Link to eLearning training via the website. There may be a cost if you do not have an NHS email account.

How and when to monitor and escalate care

Hazel Cowls

NMC *STANDARDS FOR PROFICIENCY FOR NURSING ASSOCIATES*

This chapter will address the following platforms and proficiencies:

Platform 1: Being an accountable practitioner

1.1   understand and act in accordance with the Code: Professional standards of practice and behaviour for nurses, midwives, and nursing associates, and fulfil all registration requirements.

Platform 3: Provide and monitor care

3.3   recognise and apply knowledge of commonly encountered mental, physical, behavioural, and cognitive health conditions when delivering care.

3.5   work in partnership with people to encourage shared decision-making, in order to support individuals, their families and carers to manage their own care when appropriate.

3.11   demonstrate the ability to recognise when a person's condition has improved or deteriorated by undertaking health monitoring. Interpret, promptly respond, share findings, and escalate as needed.

3.21   recognise how a person's capacity affects their ability to make decisions about their own care and to give or withhold consent

Annexe A: Communication and relationship management skills

4. demonstrate effective communication skills for working in professional teams.

Chapter aims

After reading this chapter you will be able to:

- Discuss the theory of clinical decision-making
- Understand your role in the wider multi-disciplinary team
- Understand your role in monitoring and escalating patient care

Introduction

In Chapter 4, you explored the purpose of assessment tools, looking at the validity and specificity of different tools used in a variety of clinical settings and fields of nursing associate practice. As an RNA, you will provide compassionate and safe care for people of all ages across different health and social care settings ensuring that you are upholding the four themes of the NMC Code (NMC, 2018). For example, you may be caring for children attending an acute assessment unit with their parents, or care for those living with dementia, the elderly, or people at the end of their life. As you are providing and monitoring care you will be working in partnership not only with the wider clinical team but also with people, families, and carers. You may need to look at a person's social circumstances and their environment, adding further detail to their patient's story, enabling you to make sound judgements and clinical decisions.

In this chapter, you will explore the theory of clinical reasoning and clinical decision-making. As you continually develop your knowledge and experience, you will begin to recognise when it is necessary to refer to others for reassessment and become involved in the ongoing care. You will consider your role within the wider multi-disciplinary team and review communication tools that will enable you to escalate care.

Understanding decision-making

Decision-making is about the choices we make whether that influences our every activity to dealing with or managing more complex situations.

Think about the choices you have made this morning. You may have had to decide how to travel to your work or place of study, you may have had to choose which clothes to wear today, or maybe you have discussed who would visit a family member in hospital. But what factors influence our decision-making? There are many internal and external factors that may influence our choices. For example, if you were to think about how you were going to get to work today then you may consider the weather, do you have the right clothing and footwear, can you work from home, do you have access to your own transport or do you need to use public transport and is the public transport reliable? The following factors may need to be considered before any decision-making:

- What do you hope to achieve?
- What are the choices and options available?
- What is the impact of each choice available?
- What if you were to do nothing?
- Are you relying on someone else, or does anyone else need to be informed?
- Do you have the correct equipment (if needed) and the right skills?
- Do you have time?
- Do you need to prioritise one decision over another?

These factors relate to everyday decisions that may appear to be relatively simple, but some people may find decision-making a challenge, including everyday decisions as described above. As a SNA and RNA, it is important to understand the potential negative impact having to make a choice may have on a person's health and well-being. How can you support a person who is finding it difficult to decide on a plan of action? Look at the following case study that describes a woman who is her husband's carer; she recognises the need to look after herself, but she is reluctant to decide which day to book a carer who can sit with her husband.

Case study 5.1: Jay (Part 1)

Jay is 64 years old and lives with his wife Farida. Jay was diagnosed with multiple sclerosis 20 years ago. He used intermittent catheterisation for about five years and was then fitted with a long-term indwelling urinary catheter in situ that is changed regularly as per local protocol. Farida supports Jay, helping him with washing and dressing as needed and attending appointments to meet healthcare professionals. Farida has reported that the relationship with her husband has altered slightly as she is his carer, adding that she feels exhausted and stressed. She feels guilty if she arranges something to do without her husband. Farida knows that she needs to look after herself, but she is struggling to book a day when the carer can sit with her husband. Farida acknowledges that she does not trust anyone else to look after Jay unless she is around to supervise. Not only is Farida worried about leaving her husband, but she is also worried about the cost.

Activity 5.1 Communication

As a SNA or RNA, how can you encourage Farida to leave her husband with a carer for part of the day so that she can enjoy some respite?

An outline answer is given at the end of this chapter.

System one and system two thinking

As humans, we learn to make decisions automatically or unconsciously based on our understanding or our intuition. This is often referred to as 'mental short cuts' or 'rules of thumb' or heuristics. For example, do you follow a cake recipe to the letter, or do you interpret and replace some ingredients with another ingredient? The term *'heuristic'* derived from the Greek *heuriskein*, which means 'to discover'. Early studies of heuristics were conducted during the early 1970s by psychologists Kahneman and Tversky. Heuristics are a method of discovery, or a process used for problem solving that requires limited mental effort. But this may lead to poor or inappropriate decision-making (Wastell and Howarth, 2022).

Understanding the theory

System one and system two thinking

Kahneman (2011) explains decision-making in more detail in terms of system one and system two thinking. System one thinking is fast, unconscious, automatic and is used in everyday decisions but prone to error. In contrast, system two thinking is slow, conscious, deliberate, intentional, and useful when making complex decisions. To illustrate system one and two thinking, look at the following two calculations. The first calculation is $2 \times 2 = 4$. We know this is correct and this is based on prior learning and knowledge. This is system one thinking that is fast and automatic. The second calculation is more complex and is likely to take longer to calculate $275 \times 386 =$? How are you working out this calculation, with or without a calculator? The answer is 106,500. This is system two thinking that is slow, conscious, and deliberate thinking.

Understanding clinical reasoning and clinical decision-making

We can look back to the 'founder of modern nursing', Florence Nightingale, who recognised that if people washed their hands this would help control and reduce levels of infection during the Crimean War. The process of judgement and clinical decision-making is something that all nursing professionals will experience every day and as they develop their skills and competencies, the process will become easier, and they will be able to manage more complex situations. Understanding clinical reasoning and clinical decision-making in nursing theory, practice and education has been widely researched (Nibbelink and Brewer, 2018).

Let us first explore the underpinning theory of decision-making as understanding this will enable us to apply it to various contexts. Theories of judgement and decision-making have been developed into three distinctive categories.

Understanding the theory

Normative, prescriptive, and descriptive decision-making

Normative – concentrates on how decisions should be made in an ideal world. Decision-making is viewed as rational and logical and will focus on statistics and outcomes. In health care, normative theory provides a structured approach to making rational, ethical and evidence-based decisions.

Prescriptive – examines how people make decisions and helps people to make the best choice for them. In health care, the use of National Clinical Guidelines will aid decision-making. Whilst an intuitive or humanistic model may fit into this category, individual registered nurses and RNAs gain knowledge and skills.

Descriptive – describes how people make judgements and make decisions. Focuses on real world content. The hypothetico-deductive model is an example of this category, whereby individuals gather information either before the patient encounter or other qualitative or quantitative data.

During your working day you will be gathering information, interpreting the information, and reaching a working nursing diagnosis, rather like detective work *(descriptive theory)*. This is clinical reasoning; it is a core skill that is essential to providing high-quality and safe effective patient care. You may also compare clinical reasoning to completing a jigsaw, as we tend to start with the edges of a jigsaw and then fill in the gaps in the middle. The edges of the jigsaw represent the person's story (clinical history) and the pieces in the middle are diagnostic tests, clinical assessments, and clinical guidelines that inform the clinician of the most appropriate and clinically effective interventions. Clinical reasoning is also described as clinical judgement (deciding what is wrong with a person) and clinical decision-making (deciding what to do) (Levett-Jones et al., 2010) (see Figure 5.1). Clinical reasoning plays a critical role in assessment and monitoring of patient care and patient safety. This core skill is essential to safe patient care, yet the definition of clinical reasoning has been conceptualised by healthcare professionals in multiple ways (Huesmann et al., 2023). For example, when defining clinical reasoning, nurses and nursing students offer a patient-centred view of clinical reasoning compared to other healthcare professionals, who viewed patients as passive participants of clinical reasoning (Young et al., 2018).

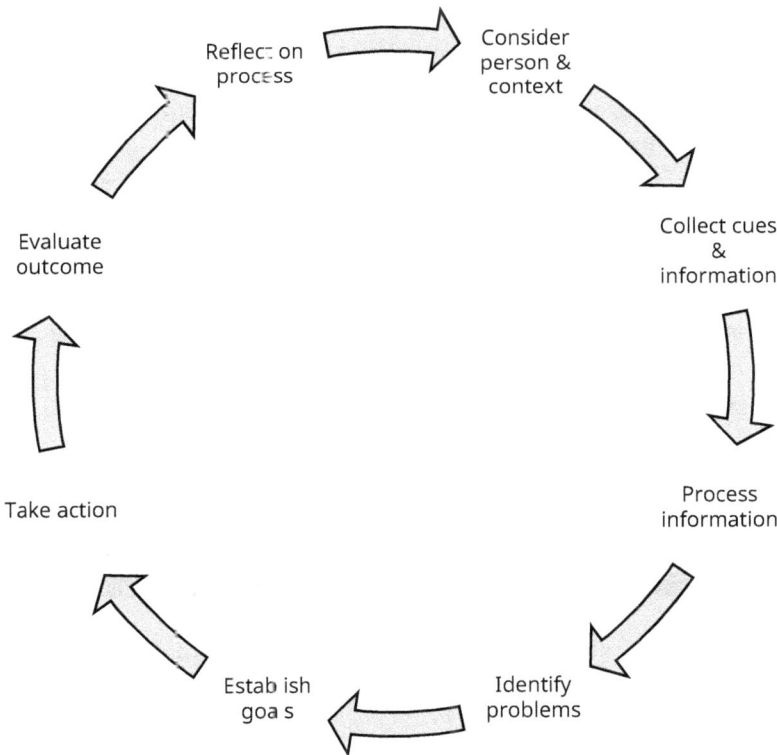

Figure 5.1 Clinical reasoning cycle

Adapted from Levett-Jones et al, 2010 (Elsevier)

The 'five rights' of clinical reasoning

The *'five rights'* of clinical reasoning provide a framework for registered nurses, RNAs, and other healthcare professionals to approach situations in a systematic manner. The five rights are as follows:

1. Right cues – able to collect accurate and relevant patient data through observation, physical examination, and history-taking.
2. Right action – implement interventions based on the cues obtained.
3. Right patient – ensuring that care provided is tailored to the individual patient.
4. Right time – being responsive and acting promptly to ensure safe patient care.
5. Right reason – being able to understand the rationale behind every clinical decision and intervention including the evidence-based practice and clinical judgement.

Let us return to Jay mentioned earlier in the chapter and apply the five rights of clinical reasoning.

Case study 5.2 Jay (Part 2)

Lillian, an RNA working in the community, has arranged to see Jay to review whether a urinary catheter change is needed.

Right cues – Jay has a long-term indwelling urinary catheter in situ that is changed regularly as per local protocol.

Right action – On this occasion, Lillian explains that a catheter change is required and obtains verbal consent from Jay. Lillian is competent in the procedure and care of catheterisation and the urinary catheter was inserted using sterile equipment and an aseptic non-touch technique (ANTT) as per local policy.

Right patient – Care provided is person-centred and verbal consent obtained and documented.

Right time – Lillian provided Jay and his wife, Farida, with after-care instructions and left.

Right reason – All possible measures must be taken to eliminate the need for catheterisation, including consideration of workable alternatives, before a decision is made to introduce a new catheter into a patient.

Activity 5.2   Reflection

Using the clinical reasoning cycle, reflect on a time when you monitored patient care and then escalated their care. Consider the following:

1. The person
2. How you collected the information
3. What problems did you identify?
4. What where the patient goals?
5. What where the interventions?
6. What was your evaluation of the situation?

As this activity is based on your own observation, there is no outline answer at the end of the chapter.

Intuition or analytical thinking

As a SNA or RNA, is your clinical reasoning and decision-making guided by recognition of patterns of behaviour or experiences or through analytical thinking? Intuition is described as the ability to understand something instinctively without any conscious reasoning (Collins Dictionary n.d.). Intuition originates from the Latin word 'intuitio', a contemplation or 'intuer', meaning to gaze upon. But how would you describe intuition? Is it a *gut feeling* or a 'sixth sense'? Something that is difficult to articulate but you recognise patterns or behaviours based on prior experience or 'tacit' knowledge (implicit knowledge) with little or no underlying conscious process and no tangible explanation. Historically, nurses' intuition was not recognised as a valid approach to decision-making as it lacked in scientific evidence (Hams, 2000). However, tacit knowledge or intuition may lead to actions on your part, such as moving a person to a clear line of sight on the ward, so that you can observe more closely as you have concerns about their well-being. This suggests that knowledge and prior experience are a core component of intuition (Benner, 1984). Rather than being viewed as a feeling, intuition could contribute to clinical reasoning decision-making.

Activity 5.3   Critical thinking

Think about clinical practice. Can you identify 'intuitive' decision-making? Describe the incident and the options available. What was the outcome of your decision-making? Positive or negative?

Although this activity is based on your own observation, there is a response at the end of the chapter.

Cognitive continuum theory

Rather than viewing intuition and analytical thinking (critical thinking) as two opposing parts, Hammond (1981) devised the cognitive continuum theory by proposing that intuition and analysis are two ends of a spectrum, and that clinical decision-making will occur somewhere along the continuum depending on the complexity of the situation. The cognitive continuum theory was revised in 2008 to provide an awareness of the multiple cognitive data that are available to nurses when making decisions. Table 5.1 below illustrates the different stages of the cognitive continuum theory ranging from intuitive or reflective judgement to scientific experiment.

Table 5.1   Revised Cognitive Continuum Theory (Standing, 2008)

Stage of Theory
Experimental research
Survey research
Qualitative research
Action research and clinical audit
Critical review of experiential research

(Continued)

Table 5.1   (Continued)

Stage of Theory
System aided judgement
Patient and peer aided judgement
Reflective judgement
Intuitive judgement

Novice to expert

As you continue to develop your clinical knowledge and practice you will move through different stages of knowledge and skills acquisition. Dreyfus (1981) named each stage as novice, advanced beginner, competent, proficient, and expert. In the novice stage, people follow directions and rules, with competence developing after exposure and significant learning. Proficiency refers to skills and intuition to make decisions and an expert can make decisions autonomously and with confidence. This model was later adopted by Benner (1982, 1984) to explain skills acquisition within nursing practice.

According to Benner (1982), a novice is described as someone who has no experience of the situation and will require demonstration as well as supervision completing tasks. An advanced beginner will be able to demonstrate some knowledge and skills and will occasionally require some support. Competency is described as the ability to do something successfully and efficiently. In nursing practice, a competent registered nurse or registered nursing associate is a person who has experience and can demonstrate efficiency and coordinated patient care. A proficient nurse or nursing associate will see the wider picture when it comes to practice, rather than individual tasks, and will be able to recognise when further intervention is required to manage a situation. Finally, the expert registered nurse or registered nursing associate will have a comprehensive understanding of any situation, and their performance will be highly proficient and skilled (Benner, 1984). Although both Dreyfus and Benner models have been criticised for the apparent linear view of knowledge and skills acquisition, the models are commonly referred to in clinical education settings.

Earlier in the chapter, we referred to Kahneman (2011) who explained system one and system two thinking that can also be applied to nursing practice. For example, as a SNA if you noticed someone clutching their chest, immediately you would think this person is uncomfortable and in pain. This would influence your actions, whether that is asking the person if they need help, calling for medical assistance, or calling for an ambulance. This is intuitive thinking (system one) that is likely to be based on experience or knowledge. In comparison, imagine you are working in an emergency department, and an ambulance crew arrives with an elderly person who was found in a collapsed state in a local shopping centre. This scenario requires slow, conscious, and analytical thinking (system two) as you and other members of the team work through an ABCDE approach to assess and treat the person (resus.org, 2024). The acronym ABCDE stands for Airway, Breathing, Circulation, Disability, Exposure and is recognised as a systematic way of assessing a person's vital signs and is particularly useful in the acute setting for assessing a deteriorating patient. The ABCDE approach is recognised as a systematic way of assessing a person's vital signs and is particularly useful in the acute setting for assessing a deteriorating patient. Vital signs are assessed in the following order, airway, breathing, circulation, disability, and exposure (see Table 5.2).

Table 5.2   ABCDE approach (resus.org, 2024)

Vital signs to check	Assessments to carry out
Airway	Look for signs of airway obstruction
	Treat as a medical emergency
	Is the patient able to speak to you?
Breathing	Is the person breathing?
	Look, listen, and feel
	Count respiratory rate
	Check patient colour
Circulation	Look, listen, and feel
	Check temperature and colour
	Check relevant vital signs
	pules and blood pressure
Disability	Is the person conscious?
	Is the person in pain?
	What is the person's blood glucose level?
	ACVPU (alert, new confusion, responds to voice, responds to pain, and unresponsive)
Exposure	Is there anything else?
	Maintaining the person's dignity, expose the person to check for other clinical signs

Understanding your role in the wider multi-disciplinary team

As a SNA and RNA, you will work in partnership with people, to encourage shared decision-making, to support individuals, their families and carers to manage their own care when appropriate. You will also need to demonstrate the necessary knowledge and skills to meet people's needs and manage their care safely, escalating care appropriately if required. Your ability to communicate with services users and colleagues is integral to your role to ensure safe, compassionate care is delivered. Remember that you are not working alone, but with a team of people across various settings to achieve a common goal. Your team is not only the people you speak to each day but could also include a wider team of people if you need to refer someone to a specialist service, for example.

Good teamwork is defined as 'the combined actions of a group of people working together effectively to achieve a goal' (Cambridge University Press, 2025) and this is essential in health and social care, but why do think teamwork is important? The principles of effective teamwork are having clear, shared objectives, working interdependently (working closely together) and meeting regularly to review their performance. The benefits of teamwork are primarily about working collaboratively with others to ensure safe patient care, as each member of the team will bring different knowledge and skills that may be required. It also provides an opportunity for people to share their knowledge and learn from each other. This, in turn, will reduce any patient harm or incident and prevent patient complaints. In addition, teamwork is about motivating each other to develop their knowledge and skills or supporting each other when required.

However, teamwork does not just happen; we all have to work together to develop a team. The following skills will enable you to work effectively and collaboratively within a team.

- Effective listening skills
- Excellent communication skills
- Effective time management skills
- Assertiveness skills
- Able to give feedback
- Able to receive feedback from others
- Able to delegate work
- Reflective practice – identifying what has gone well, what you have learnt and what could be improved
- Problem-solving skills
- Situational awareness
- Emotional intelligence – the ability to identify your own emotion and how others are feeling

Let us return to Jay mentioned earlier in the chapter and apply the ABCDE approach.

Case study 5.3: Jay (Part 3)

Unfortunately, Jay has been admitted to the emergency room due to increasing dyspnoea at rest. The nurse in charge asks Stefan (RNA) to complete a set of vital signs and report the results to the admitting doctor. Stefan introduces himself to Jay, explaining their role and obtains verbal consent to complete a set of vital signs. Jay is struggling to talk in full sentences, but Stefan has established that Jay has been feeling generally unwell for approximately 48 hours, but this morning he felt worse, and his wife called an ambulance.

Stefan completes Jay's vital signs and is concerned about Jay's health; Stefan explains to Jay that they are going to call the doctor to request an urgent review. Stefan was feeling worried as this was their first day in the emergency department and had limited experience of working in an acute setting. However, Stefan needs to remain calm and professional so as not to worry Jay. Stefan contacted the doctor and hands over the following:

Airway – open as Jay can talk
Breathing – visibly breathless, respiratory rate 24, pulse oximetry 90 per cent on air
Circulation – pulse 120 bpm, regular, blood pressure 100/60
Disability – capillary blood glucose 5.2 mmol, (ACVPU) (see Table 5.2) alert, no new confusion
Exposure – no wounds, no fluid loss, temperature 37.9 Celsius

Stefan waits for instructions from the doctor and informs the nurse in charge.

This final part of Jay's care illustrates good listening skills as Stefan takes time to listen to Jay's story. Stefan was self-aware and knew that they needed to remain calm and professional, demonstrating emotional intelligence. Emotional intelligence refers to the ability to manage situations and communicate effectively with others. Stefan identifies that Jay is unwell and needs an urgent clinical review, so they complete Jay's vital signs and prepare to hand them over to the doctor demonstrating good communication skills, assertive skills, and situational awareness.

As an RNA it is important to continually develop clinical skills and communication skills to ensure high-quality safe patient care is a priority. This is achieved through reflective practice and obtaining feedback from your colleagues and peers.

Registered nurse associate voice

The below quote is from a Registered Nursing Associate speaking about her role within the community nursing team.

I feel supported by the team, and we all work together to provide safe, good quality care. I find having my own caseload is empowering.

Activity 5.4   Reflection

Good teamwork is essential when we are providing patient care and equally important is the ability to delegate work as well as giving and receiving feedback. Think about a time when you delegated work or either gave or received feedback to another person. You may wish to use the following reflective model (Gibbs, 1988):

1.   Describe the situation
2.   How did you feel?
3.   What was good and bad about the situation?
4.   What sense can you make of the situation?
5.   What have you learnt and what could you do better?
6.   What is your action plan?

As this activity is based on your own observation, there is no outline answer at the end of the chapter.

The benefits of working in a team are improved patient outcomes and higher quality personalised care. The following scenarios will illustrate how you can show that you are working collaboratively with others (NMC, 2018). For the first, keep the 'jigsaw' analogy mentioned earlier in this chapter in mind.

Case study 5.4: Working collaboratively with others in an outpatient clinic

Imagine that you are the SNA running an outpatient clinic, a patient is attending a fracture clinic. You introduce yourself to the patient and obtain verbal consent to collect information that may help identify the patient's needs. You gather information that includes the patient's demographic details, social history, occupation history, and medication history. The patient reports ongoing pain, and they have limited movement in their left arm. You may ask them

(Continued)

for more details about the injury. You realise that the patient needs further tests so refer to a doctor based in the department. You hand over the essential information to the doctor. The doctor reviews the patient and requests an X-ray of their left arm. The doctor prescribes some medication to ease the patient's pain.

This scenario illustrates the five rights in clinical reasoning. The SNA gathers patient specific information *(right cues)*, the SNA speaks with the medical team *(right action)* immediately *(right time)* to ensure the patient has access to individualised *(right patient)* and evidence-based care *(right reason)*. In accordance with the NMC standards for Nursing Associates the case study illustrates the SNA is working collaboratively with others (Standard 4.1) and able to prioritise and delegate care appropriately if needed (Standard 4.5).

Case study 5.5: Working collaboratively with others on a cardiology ward

You are an RNA working on a cardiology ward, and you are supervising an SNA. The student asked that you observe them recording an electrocardiogram (ECG) and that you give them feedback on their practice. You observe the student introducing themselves to the patient and explaining the procedure. The student obtains consent and ensures the patient's dignity is maintained throughout the procedure. The student records an ECG (as per local guidelines), dates and signs the ECG and places in the patient records for review from the medical team.

You provide feedback as requested, highlighting good practice and any areas for improvement.

In this scenario, the RNA supports the SNA (NMC, 2024, Standard 4.2) by providing constructive feedback to a colleague when care has been delegated (NMC, 2024, Standard 4.6). The RNA is also acting as a role model to nursing students, health care support workers, and people that are new to care roles (NMC, Standard 4.7).

Activity 5.4   Reflection

Review platform 4 of the Standards of Proficiency for Nursing Associates (NMC, 2024), choose one of the standards and reflect on a time when you have demonstrated that skill. For example, can you recall a time when you were able to support and motivate a member of the care team and interact confidently with them.

As this activity is based on your own observation, there is no outline answer at the end of the chapter.

Tools for monitoring and escalating patient care

As a SNA and RNA, you will make simple and complex decisions every day that will affect patient care. This will range from carrying out and recording a person's blood pressure to a team of people deciding the best treatment for someone who is newly diagnosed with a life-limiting illness. Regardless of whether the decision-making is simple or complex you will go through a process to ensure that care is safe, person-centred and effective. Remember good decisions equal safe patient care.

In Chapter 4, you reviewed the purpose of assessment tools and to understand the validity and specificity of different tools used in various clinical settings and fields of nursing associate practice. You will recognise the importance of using assessment tools in practice to support your clinical decision-making. The ABCDE Approach (resus.org, 2024) mentioned earlier in the chapter is a systematic process for assessing and monitoring people who may be acutely unwell and can be useful when combined with other communication tools to escalate patient care. The ability to speak up and express concern about the health and well-being of an individual is an essential skill for staff working in health and social care settings. There are a few recognised communication tools (acronyms) that support an effective handover of care.

SBARD

The first one is the SBARD approach (situation, background, assessment, recommendation, decision) communication tool. SBARD tool is an effective tool for communicating a handover of care or for escalating care. The World Health Organization (2007) recommends the use of SBAR as a tool to standardise handover communications, although they acknowledge that one system or tool may not suit all clinical settings and that local adaptations may be needed. Prior to handing over care, you need to gather information to present succinctly to another person.

Situation – introduce oneself, explain the situation, your concern, and who is involved.

Background – provide specific information about the person involved (name, age, medical history, medication, and clinical observations).

Assessment – explain the problem, what you have done, or what your concern is.

Recommendation – what do you want to happen and what can you do in the meantime.

Decision – repeat back and document any plan.

RSVP

The second approach is the RVSP approach (Reason, Story, Vital signs, Plan).

Reason – introduce oneself and your reason for escalating patient care.

Story – share background information.

Vital Signs – explain the current problem and report the current patient vital signs.

Plan – agree a plan.

Case study 5.7: Sam (Part 1)

Nursing Associate Davies is working on a children's admission ward and looking after a six-year-old that becomes acutely ill. Following the local policy and out of concern for Sam, care is escalated to the Foundation Year 1 doctor covering the children's admission ward.

Situation – Hello Dr. This is Nursing Associate Davies. I am calling you about Sam who is six-year-old, admitted overnight with acute asthma.

Background – Sam was admitted around 10 pm last night after waking up struggling to breathe. No medical history of note. Treated with nebulised salbutamol (2.5 mg) and ipratropium bromide (250 mcg).

Assessment –This morning Sam is experiencing severe asthma, agitated and distressed, unable to talk in sentences. Heart rate is 124 beats per minute, O2 saturations on air are <92 per cent. I have applied high flow oxygen as prescribed, and a colleague is about to start nebulised salbutamol. *This is where you may add the ABCDE assessment.*

Recommendation – I am really concerned about Sam and feel that an urgent review is required.

Decision – Thank you, so just to confirm, you would like me to continually monitor Sam, and you will review in five minutes.

In Case Study 5.7, Davies can work with the doctor to agree a care plan for Sam. How would you manage a situation if you called for advice and the person you were calling decides that there is no urgency or suggests a clinical management plan that you do not think will be effective? Knowing how to speak up and raise your concern is a key safety factor (Lancman et al., 2015). If this were to occur, you could use graded assertiveness to express your concerns. PACE (probe, alert, challenge, escalate) is useful when you need to challenge any action or behaviours that may feel inappropriate or unsafe. *Probe* is about getting someone's attention or raising a concern. *Alert* is repeating your concern if you feel you do not have someone's attention. *Challenge* is to formally raise a concern and even challenge a decision made. *Escalate (or Emergency)* is to take charge and that may mean referring to someone more senior. Let us illustrate how PACE can be used by returning to the story of Sam on the child assessment unit.

Case study 5.8: Sam (Part 2)

The Foundation Year 1 doctor arrives on the ward to review Sam. You and your colleague are present and explain that you have administered nebulised salbutamol as prescribed, but you remain concerned.

Probe – thank you for coming to review Sam so quickly, I am still quite worried about their condition.

Alert – I understand that the medication can take a while to have an effect, but Sam has been feeling like this for at least 20 minutes.

Challenge – I realise that salbutamol can be repeated but they are already tachycardic and appear agitated and unable to speak. I am not happy with the decision to watch and wait.

Escalate (emergency) – do we need to call a senior medic to review Sam. Would you like me to call them?

Different approaches and tools of communication will ensure that as a SNA or RNA you provide a clear and safe escalation of care. In practice you may find it helpful to prepare your handover prior to escalation. If you are not comfortable with the decision, then ask your colleague to explain as this will help you to understand and continue to develop your knowledge and skills.

Chapter summary

This chapter has explored the theory of clinical decision-making, your role in the wider multi-disciplinary team, and your role in monitoring and escalating patient care. As a SNA and RNA, you will make clinical decisions every day, and these may include simple tasks such as supporting a patient who needs to access a bathroom to more complex decisions. SBARD, RSVP, and PACE are useful acronyms to use in practice should you need to escalate care. The case studies have provided additional information to help contextualise your role working in the wider multi-disciplinary team. The activities have provided you with an opportunity to reflect on your practice and to develop a deeper understanding of monitoring patient care.

Activities: Brief outline answers

Activity 5.1 Communication (page 73)

You may need to question why Farida is reluctant to leave her husband. Give her time to explore her worries and concerns. Find out from Farida what she wants, does she just want some time to go for a coffee with her friend or to attend a GP appointment? Offer reassurance to Farida if indicated.

Activity 5.3 Critical thinking (page 77)

It is acknowledged that practitioners are more likely to recall examples where intuition can be linked to a positive outcome. This may then confirm intuition as an effective decision-making strategy.

Further reading

Glasper (2021) Raising and escalating concerns about patient care: RCN guidance. *British Journal of Nursing*. Available at: www.britishjournalofnursing.com/content/healthcare-policy/raising-and-escalating-concerns-about-patient-care-rcn-guidance/

Huesmann, L., Sudacka, M., Durning, S. J., Georg, C., Huwendiek, S., Kononowicz, A. A., Hege, I. (2023) Clinical reasoning: What do nurses, physicians, and students reason about. *Journal of Interprofessional Care*, 37(6), 990–998. https://doi.org/10.1080/13561820.2023.2208605

Kahneman, D. (2011) *Thinking, Fast and Slow*. Doubleday Canada.

NHS England (2010) Safer Care SBAR Situation • Background • Assessment • Recommendation. Available at: www.england.nhs.uk/improvement-hub/wp-content/uploads/sites/44/2017/11/SBAR-Implementation-and-Training-Guide.pdf

Watch

Thinking Fast and Slow (Kahneman, 2011) https://youtu.be/CjVQJdIrDJo?si=qRD_o3bl2035R5Hh

Professor Michael West www.youtube.com/watch?v=bqipJlb1oMM

Useful websites

'Let's talk about professional judgement | Caring with Confidence: The Code in Action | NMC Available at: www.youtube.com/watch?v=O4IWH-w4xLA

As a nurse, midwife or nursing associate, you use your professional judgement to make decisions. An informative video from the Nursing and Midwifery Council on professional judgement.

National Early Warning Score (NEWS) 2 Available at: www.rcp.ac.uk/improving-care/resources/national-early-warning-score-news-2/

Information on NEWS2, the aggregate scoring system in which a score is allocated to physiological measurements, when patients present to, or are being monitored in hospital. Link to elearning training via the website. There may be a cost if you do not have an NHS email account.

Communication tool (SBARD) Available at: www.england.nhs.uk/improvement-hub/wp-content/uploads/sites/44/2017/11/SBAR-Implementation-and-Training-Guide.pdf

Explanation of how to escalate a deteriorating patient safely using the acronym SBARD.

Communication tool (PACE) Available at: www.pslhub.org/learn/improving-patient-safety/rcog-probe-alert-challenge-and-escalate-model-pace-r2953/

Explanation of how to use graded assertiveness when raising a concern about a person's condition.

Recognition and Management of the Sick Child Available at: https://geekymedics.com/recognition-and-management-of-the-sick-child/

Explanation of how to recognise an unwell child, how to carry out a structured A-E assessment, and how this can be adapted depending on the child's developmental age.

Paediatric Early Warning Systems (PEWS) Royal College of Paediatrics and Child Health Available at: www.rcpch.ac.uk/resources/UK-paediatric-early-warning-systems

The early warning system is designed to recognise and respond to the deteriorating child or young person.

Chapter 6

The principles and theories of planning nursing care

Hazel Cowls

> ## Chapter aims
>
> After reading this chapter you will:
>
> - Be able to explain the theory and principles of the nursing process;
> - Explore nursing models and how these support high quality, compassionate care delivery;
> - Understand how nursing models relate to the nursing associate role;
> - Understand the difference between care bundles and care pathways.

Introduction

It is important to understand the underpinning theory of the nursing process and nursing models. This chapter will introduce you to the principles of the nursing process and how this process supports your practice as an student nurse associate (SNA) and registered nurse associate (RNA). The NMC (2024) have been clear about the role of a registered nurse (RN) and RNA when it comes to assessing, planning and monitoring care (see Table 6.1). Both the RN and RNA are accountable professionals, promoting health and preventing ill health, improving quality and safety of care. You will explore how nursing models when used alongside the nursing process will ensure that care is assessed, planned, delivered, monitored, and evaluated effectively. You will be introduced to three nursing models that are the Human Needs Model (Roper, Logan and Tierney, 2000), Self-care model of nursing (Orem, 2001) and Moulster and Griffiths model (2012). You will consider how these models can be applied to your clinical practice in health and social care. You will recognise that the application of a problem-solving process (ASPIRE) and a nursing model provides a consistent comprehensive framework that will ensure care is assessed, planned, delivered, monitored, and evaluated. Finally, you will be introduced to care pathways and care bundles, explore how evidence-base improves patient outcomes and supports clinical practice in health and social care settings.

Table 6.1 Understanding the different levels of responsibility for an RNA and RN

Role	Assess	Plan	Provide and monitor	Evaluate
Registered nurse	Yes	Yes	Yes	Yes
Registered nursing associate	Contribute to care and reassessment	Contribute to planning	Yes	

The principles of the nursing process

Historically, nursing was focused on tasks and was often perceived as ritualistic practice. However, Yura and Walsh (1967) wanted to move away from intuitive ritualistic practice by providing a systematic framework that included assessment, planning, implementation, and evaluation (APIE). This process was later called the nursing process and has been defined as:

an organised, systematic, and deliberate approach to nursing with the aim of improving standards in nursing care.

Rush et al., 1996

The name suggests that only nurses can use this framework when the reality is that any healthcare professional could follow this approach (Wilson et al., 2019). Each step of the nursing process (APIE) has been described by Yura and Walsh (1967):

1. **Assessment.** This step involves data collection such as observational data, clinical signs (such as pulse, blood pressure and respiratory rate) as well as listening to the person's story to understand their presenting problem and health needs. As an SNA or RNA, you may be involved in recording or reassessing a person's vital signs, you may also need to speak with other relevant people such as a parent or carer to elicit a clear history if the person is unable to communicate.
2. **Planning.** This step involves choosing evidence-based nursing interventions that will address the person's needs. It is important to include the person in any decision-making activities ensuring a person-centred approach.
3. **Implementation.** The third step of APIE is about implementing or providing care. As an SNA or RNA, you will be actively involved in the implementation of care.
4. **Evaluation.** The final step is evaluating care delivered, for example has there been an improvement in the person's condition. As an SNA/RNA, you will be working with the multi-disciplinary team and evaluating care. Figure 6.1 illustrates the logical order of the nursing process.

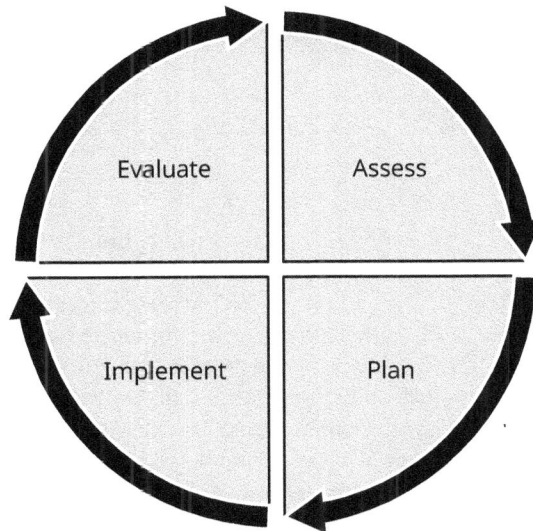

Figure 6.1 APIE: The nursing process

Source: Adapted from Wilson, Woollands and Barrett, (2019).

Wilson et al. (2019) expanded on APIE by including two additional steps that are a *systematic nursing diagnosis* and *recheck,* and APIE becomes ASPIRE (see Figure 6.2).

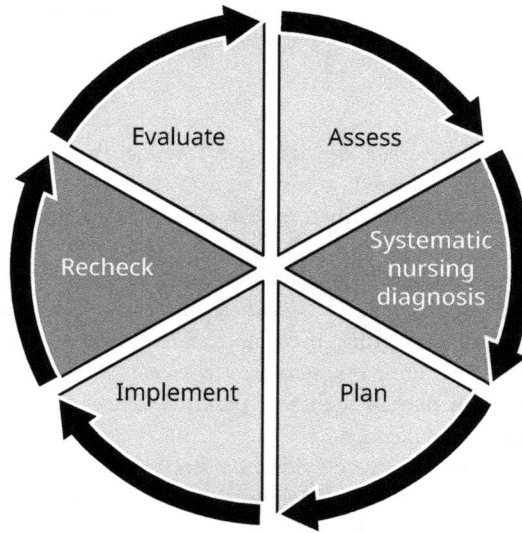

Figure 6.2 ASPIRE: a problem-solving approach

Source: adapted from Wilson, Woollands and Barrett (2019).

The first of these steps is a *'systematic nursing diagnosis'*, which ensures that the patient's needs are understood so that the nurse can identify actual or potential health problems and formulise an individual person-centred care plan. An example of a nursing diagnosis is delayed child development (or delayed milestone attainment), which is:

> a deficiency in the normal sequence of age-related milestones leading to impaired physical, cognitive, emotional, or social functioning.

Nanda.org (2024).

The diagnosis may be due to an underlying factor such as prematurity, genetic abnormality, environmental hazards, disease, or trauma. In this case, it is likely that the RN and SNA/RNA will need to liaise with the family and other healthcare professionals to coordinate care, monitor the child's progress, and implement specific interventions.

Another nursing diagnosis is insomnia, a common sleep disturbance characterised by difficulty falling asleep, staying asleep or feeling tired all day even after sleep. Insomnia is a common problem across all ages and populations. One definition of insomnia is 'disturbed sleep related to inadequate nocturnal sleep' (Nanda.org). There may be several potential reasons why a person experiences insomnia such as depression, asthma, heart failure, pain, and irregular work patterns to name a few. The registered nurse and SNA/RNA will provide specific interventions that will help people identify the cause of insomnia and improve their sleep pattern.

The second step added is *'recheck'* which precedes evaluation. This step is about gathering specific and targeted information linked to the individual's specific problem and goal. The SNA/RNA is required to describe and document the patient's present condition and progress to date; this underpins the evaluation stage. The following case study illustrates the six steps of ASPIRE.

Case study 6.1: Ronnie

Ronnie is 19 years old and has attended the GP clinic to see the RNA for routine blood tests as requested by the GP. Ronnie reports a lack of sleep and feels this is impacting on everyday life.

Using the ASPIRE framework the RNA and Ronnie agree the following:

1. **Assess** – Ronnie is struggling to get up in the morning and is frequently late for class at university.
2. **Systematic nursing diagnosis** – insomnia.
3. **Plan** – the RNA provides specific interventions about sleep hygiene practices and relaxation techniques. Examples include keeping a regular sleep/wake schedule, avoid stimulants such as caffeine, engage in regular exercise during the day and to record a sleep diary for review in two weeks.
4. **Implementation** – as discussed, Ronnie looks at steps to improve sleep hygiene and records her sleep pattern.
5. **Recheck** – at the next consultation Ronnie meets the RNA to discuss their sleep pattern over the last two weeks.
6. **Evaluation** – they both agree that there has been some improvement, although Ronnie needs to continue to reduce any drinks which contain caffeine.

In summary, ASPIRE provides a systematic framework for the delivery of person-centred nursing care, supported by nursing models or philosophies. ASPIRE ensures the SNA/RNA and rest of the nursing team along with the patient work together to problem solve and set person-centred goals. One way of looking at it is as a road map representing all the possible routes, and it is the driver's choice to choose the best route for them.

Understanding nursing models

There is a close relationship between the nursing process and nursing models, the nursing process is used to provide structure to the delivery of care and a nursing model provides additional detail to delivering care. In this section, you will understand how the nursing process and a nursing model are inextricably linked, and the case studies will provide real-world application of the theories to specific scenarios.

First, let us look at the origins of nursing models. They date back to the nineteenth century when Florence Nightingale cared for soldiers during the Crimean war. She was known for being a pioneer in modern nursing and authored several books on nursing, one of which was the foundation for the curriculum for nursing schools of the time. Mary Seacole is another inspirational nurse from the same period; however, unlike Florence Nightingale, Mary self-funded to care for soldiers during the Crimean war. Virginia Henderson (born 1897) is another influential figure and was a nurse, researcher, theorist, and writer. She is known as the 'first lady of nursing' and her written work has been viewed as the twentieth-century equivalent of work from the founder of modern nursing, Florence Nightingale (Halloran, 1996). Virginia Henderson wrote about the basic principles and practice of nursing and developed one of the first nursing theories. Henderson identified three main beliefs in her model:

1. The nurse will care for a 'patient' until he or she can care for themselves.
2. The nurse will care for a 'patient' day and night.
3. The nurse will be educated at the college level in both sciences and arts.

Henderson (1969) also identified 14 components based on human needs that make up nursing interventions, ranging from physical needs to psychological and social needs.

1. Breathe normally.
2. Eat and drink adequately.
3. Eliminate body wastes.
4. Move and maintain desirable postures.
5. Sleep and rest.
6. Select suitable clothing.
7. Maintain body temperature within normal range by adjusting clothing and modifying the environment.
8. Keep the body clean and well-groomed.
9. Avoid dangers in the environment and avoid injuring others.
10. Communicate with others.
11. Worship according to one's faith.
12. Work.
13. Play or recreational activity.
14. Continue to learn, discover, that leads to normal development and health.

Nursing models attempt to organise the process of nursing care and in doing so ensure that there is consistency in understanding what care is needed, when patients are unable to provide for their own needs, and how this care should be carried out. Nursing models have been described as 'conceptual tools that can be used by an individual to understand and place complex phenomena into perspective' (McKenna, 1997, p. 12). The three basic components of a contemporary nursing model are:

1. A view of the person's beliefs and values.
2. A statement on the goal of nursing.
3. A statement on the knowledge and skills required by the nurse.

To explain this further, Table 6.2 illustrates three nursing models and each of the components; these models will be discussed in more detail.

Table 6.2   Components of three nursing models

Model	Views of the person	Goal of nursing	Knowledge and skills of the nurse
Human Needs Model (Roper, Logan and Tierney, 2000)	12 Activities of daily living (ADLs) over the lifespan.	Help people to prevent or solve actual or potential problems related to the 12 ADLs.	Understanding of the biopsychosocial, environmental and political factors that may impact on the 12 ADLs.
Self-care model (Orem, 2001)	All individuals have the capacity for self-care.	To help individuals overcome any deficits in self-care due to ill health.	Promotion of self-care through guidance, support and teaching.
Moulster and Griffiths (2009)	Enabling people at risk of exclusion due to age or disability to live a life as they choose.	To empower people to live as equal citizens and take a lead in decision making.	To implement best practice and promote inclusion and equality.

Human needs model

Roper, Logan and Tierney's Human Needs Model (1980) was based on Henderson's needs model (1969) and was developed as a conceptual framework to introduce nursing students to individualised person-centred care (Tierney, 2020). There are five key components to this model:

1. Twelve activities of daily living.
2. Five influencing factors.
3. Lifespan continuum.
4. Independence/Dependence continuum.
5. Individuality.

The twelve activities of daily living (ADLs) are listed below and will be explored in more detail.

1. Maintaining a safe environment.
2. Communication.
3. Breathing.
4. Eating and drinking.
5. Elimination.
6. Personal cleansing and dressing.
7. Controlling body temperature.
8. Mobilising.
9. Working and playing.
10. Expressing sexuality.
11. Sleeping.
12. Dying.

The five influencing factors are:

1. Biological – influenced by a person's overall health.
2. Psychological – influenced by factors such as intellect, emotional factors, cognition, and spiritual beliefs.
3. Sociocultural – influenced by belief systems such as values that are based on social class or status.
4. Environmental – influenced by the environment but also the person's effect on the environment.
5. Political – influenced by governments, national, and local policies.

The model can be used across the lifespan and provides a framework when assessing a patient; you have probably noted that it includes the bio-psycho-social and spiritual needs of a person as discussed in Chapter 3. The model should not be used as a checklist, but rather a continuous assessment of a person's dependence and independence. Continually assessing a person's dependence and independence will allow the nurse or SNA/RNA to determine whether a person is improving or deteriorating. For example, a person is admitted to hospital with pneumonia and reports no previous problems with their breathing (usual state) but describes symptoms of struggling to walk upstairs or steps and at rest (current state). This model has been widely adopted in the United Kingdom and Ireland in general settings, intensive care settings (Robb, 1997), as well as neonatal units (O'Connor and Timmins, 2002), often used as a preliminary assessment of patient needs.

Activity 6.1   Critical thinking

Choose one of the five influencing factors from the Human Needs model and describe why this is important when you are providing and monitoring patient care.

An outline answer is given at the end of this chapter.

Case study 6.2: Sam

Sam is a 58-year-old admitted to hospital with a recent history of numbness, an inability to move their left arm or leg, difficulty speaking, difficulty swallowing and a headache. Sam is currently on medication for hypertension (high blood pressure). Using the Human Needs model (Roper, Logan and Tierney, 1980) an initial assessment of daily living is carried out. Table 6.3 illustrates A of ASPIRE.

Table 6.3   Activities of daily living

Activities of daily living	Usual state	Current state
Maintaining a safe environment	Able to maintain own safe environment	Unable to maintain a safe environment
Communication	Usually independent, no hearing aids, wears reading glasses	Difficulty speaking. May require aids to communicate while in hospital.
Breathing	No problems identified	No problems identified
Eating and drinking	No problems identified, eats a vegetarian diet	Difficulty swallowing
Elimination	Normal bowel movements	May require assistance to access toilet facilities.
Personal cleansing and dressing	Independent	Not independent
Controlling body temperature	Independent	Not independent
Mobilising	Independent, no aids required	Left-sided weakness, not able to weight bear
Working and playing	Employed and active	Currently in hospital and limited mobility
Expressing sexuality	Heterosexual Self-image	Not independent
Sleeping	Usually takes herbal medication to aid sleep.	Sleep may be disturbed while in hospital.
Dying	Independent	May express thoughts of dying while in hospital.

As an SNA/RNA, you may not be involved in the initial patient assessment, but you will be involved in continually assessing the patient's current state. For example, if we were to look at the first six ADLs illustrated in Sam's case study, the continuing assessment, providing and monitoring of care would look like the following (Table 6.4):

Table 6.4 Activities of daily living: reassessment and monitoring of care (of 6 ADLs)

Activities of daily living	Current state	SNA/RNA role
Maintaining a safe environment	Unable to maintain a safe environment.	Monitor Sam's vital signs and report any deterioration.
Communication	Difficulty speaking. May require aids to communicate while in hospital.	Ensure Sam's reading glasses are available to aid reading.
		Use visual boards to aid communication.
		Report any deterioration.
Breathing	No problems identified.	Monitor respiratory rate as part of assessment of vital signs.
		Report any deterioration.
Eating and drinking	Difficulty swallowing	Check a referral to the speech and language therapist (SALT) for a swallow assessment has been made.
Elimination	May require assistance to access toilet facilities.	Provide assistance if required.
		Maintain Sam's dignity.
Personal cleansing and dressing	Not independent	Provide assistance if required.
		Maintain Sam's dignity.

Self-care model

Orem's self-care model consists of three interrelated theories: self-care; self-care deficit; and nursing system (see Figure 6.3). Self-care is based around the nurse's assessment of a person's own ability to maintain health and well-being. The theory of self-care deficit is where the nurse confirms the needs and limitations of the person. Once this has been confirmed, a member of the nursing team will consider five methods of helping: acting, guiding, physical and psychological support, and promotion of health needs and teaching. The final component is the theory of nursing systems, which considers the role of the nurse and the nursing associate. There are three nursing system classifications to meet the self-care needs of the person:

- Wholly compensatory system – the person needs complete care.
- Partial compensatory system – some limitations but able to perform some self-care requisites independently.
- Supportive-educative – independent and requires education to promote self-care.

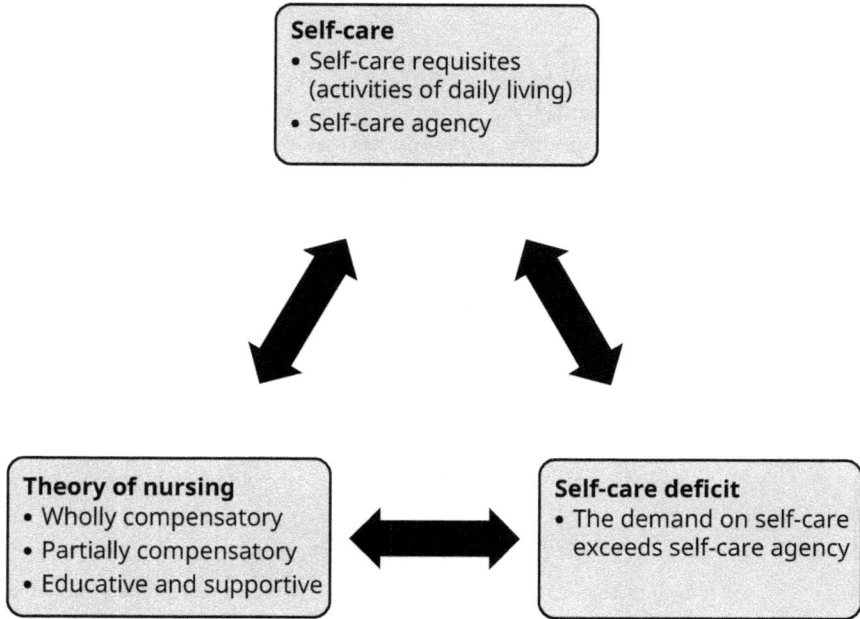

Figure 6.3   Orem self-care model

This model can also be applied to the role of the SNA/RNA as illustrated in the case study below.

Case study 6.3: Remy

Remy is six years old and while at school he experiences an exacerbation of asthma. Remy is taken to see the school nursing team, the SNA telephones Remy's mother. Remy's mother agrees that Remy should return to see the school nursing team in one month, to review how Remy is self-managing symptoms.

Self-care – Remy is independent with self-care requisites.

Self-care deficit – Remy stated that he sometimes feels breathless when he is playing sports or running around outside at breaktime.

Nursing system (Educative and supportive) – Through supportive, educative play the SNA can provide Remy with information on how he can manage his symptoms to become competent in their self-care.

Moulster and Griffiths model

In Chapter 3, you were introduced to the role of the learning disability nurse and how to meet the biopsychosocial (BPS) needs for someone with a learning disability. The Moulster and Griffiths model (2009) was developed to meet the needs of people with a learning disability and to support learning disability nursing. The model clarifies the role of the learning disability nurses, ensuring that all people with a learning disability have access to care that is person-centred, and evidence based. This model was developed in 2009 and refers to the nursing process (APIE – assessment, planning, implementation, and evaluation). There are seven stages to this model as it guides nurses to complete assessments, plan care based on evidence-based interventions and reflective evaluations. The model does draw on elements from Orem's (2001) self-care model, Aldridge's (2004) person-centred ecology of health for people with learning disability, McCormack and McCance's (2006) outcome-focused, person-centred framework as well as Gibbs' (1988) reflective model and a health equality framework (HEF) (Atkinson et al., 2013). As previously discussed in Chapter 3, people with a learning disability will experience poorer health and live in poor housing; the health equality framework is an aggregation tool that measures the wider determinants of health for people with a learning disability (Atkinson et al., 2015). Table 6.5 illustrates the elements of this model.

Table 6.5 The nursing process (APIE) and Moulster and Griffiths model

Stages		Additional elements
Nursing Process	Moulster & Griffiths model	
Assessment	1. Person-centred	Reflection
	2. Nursing assessment	
	3. HEF	
Planning	4. Nursing care plan	Evidence-based
		Reflection
Implementation	5 Nursing implementation	Reflection
Evaluation	6. Care plan evaluation	Reflection
	7 HEF evaluation	

Source: Adapted from Moulster et al. (2019).

The following case study illustrates the seven steps of the Moulster and Griffiths model.

Case study 6.4 Aubrey

Aubrey is 22 years old and has moderate learning disability. Aubrey was referred to the community learning disability nursing team for lifestyle education after concerns over their lifestyle and family environment Aubrey has recently been diagnosed with diabetes.

Assessment (to be carried out by the community learning disability nurse)

The community learning disability nurse assessed Aubrey; their uncle was also present at the initial assessment. An SNA was observing the assessment. Initially, Aubrey was reluctant to speak; however, as he relaxed Aubrey spoke about what was important to him, such as his mixed African and European heritage. Aubrey had recently moved into sheltered accommodation but appeared to be struggling to manage his finances. Aubrey was obese, took little exercise, was unaware of healthy eating and a smoker. Aubrey did not speak of any friends and appeared isolated from a family environment.

The HEF score showed that without intervention, Aubrey's health and well-being is at risk of deteriorating.

(Continued)

Care plan *(to be agreed with Aubrey)*

The community learning disability nurse and SNA helped Aubrey create an easy-read care plan based on their aspirations, which were to:

- speak to GP or practice nurse about stopping smoking;
- to join an exercise class or walking group;
- to find out about healthy eating;
- to spend more time with family.

Implementation *(review by SNA under supervision)*

The SNA arranges to revisit Aubrey in one week to review progress.

At the next visit, Aubrey states that the GP had referred him to the stop smoking service and he had been prescribed Nicotine replacement therapy. Aubrey states that he still has the urge to smoke but has not since commencing nicotine replacement therapy. Aubrey has attended an assessment at a local exercise group and enjoyed the first session. Aubrey is thinking about healthy eating and eating more fruits and vegetables. Aubrey has arranged to visit his uncle at the weekend.

Evaluation *(completed by community learning disability nurse and SNA)*

Aubrey's HEF score has decreased, reflecting improvements in their lifestyle. A recommendation is made for a three-month check-up with the SNA or another member of the learning disability team as well as an annual check-up appointment with the GP.

Reflection *(completed by community learning disability nurse and SNA)*

In their reflection, the community learning disability nurse and SNA were able to identify key domains in Aubrey's care where nursing interventions had made a difference.

According to the Public Health Observatory (Emerson and Baines, 2011) there are five determinants of health that are commonly experienced by people with a learning disability. These are:

1. Social determinants;
2. Genetic and biological determinants;
3. Communication difficulties and reduced health literacy;
4. Personal health behaviour and lifestyle risks;
5. Deficiencies in access to and quality of health provision.

In Aubrey's case study, they may have some communication difficulties and reduced health literacy, lifestyle risks and possibly reduced access to health provision.

Activity 6.2 Research

You have looked at three contemporary nursing models. Please research either Family-centred care (Casey, 1988) used in children's nursing, or the Tidal Model commonly used in mental health nursing (Barker and Buchanan-Barker, 2005) and answer the following questions.

1. What are the views of the person's beliefs and values?
2. What is the goal of nursing?
3. What knowledge and skills are required by you as the nursing associate?

An outline answer is given at the end of this chapter.

Care bundles and care pathways

The purpose of care bundles and care pathways is to ensure that all patients/clients/service users across the United Kingdom have access to evidence-based care by providing a systematic framework to guide clinicians. The concept of a care bundle was first explored in 2001 and defined as:

> *small set of evidence-based interventions for a defined patient segment/population and care setting that, when implemented together, will result in significantly better outcomes than when implemented individually.*

> Resar et al., 2001, p. 2.

Care bundles

A care bundle is a structured way of improving care and patient outcomes. It uses a small set of evidence-based interventions (generally 3–5) that have been proven to be shown to be beneficial to patient care individually. A 'bundle' ties these interventions together, the idea being that implementing them together will result in better outcomes than when they're used alone – all the interventions need to be used in a care bundle, rather than completing for example, three out of the four steps.

So, how does a care bundle differ from a checklist? Care bundles are based on randomised controlled trials that are accepted and well established. The bundle focuses on how to deliver the best care based on the best evidence by completing each step. All healthcare professionals, including RNAs, are expected to complete any relevant care bundle documentation so that all members of the team are aware which steps have been completed. A checklist, on the other hand, is a list of processes that need to be completed – for example the World Health Organization (WHO) surgical checklist. The WHO surgical checklist is completed at three separate times:

Sign in – completed before anaesthesia and in the presence of the anaesthetist.

Time out – completed before the first incision; final opportunity to identify the patient, the procedure, and the site involved.

Sign out – completed prior to key members of the operating team leaving the operating room.

There are many care bundles seen in clinical practice. One example is the sepsis six care bundle that was produced by the UK Sepsis Trust along with the National Institute for Health and Care Excellence (NICE). The sepsis care bundle is six tasks that if implemented within one hour or less with improve a person's clinical outcome (NICE, 2024) (see Table 6.6).

Table 6.6   Sepsis six care bundle

Action	Time	Initials
Ensure senior clinicians reviews patient		
Give oxygen if required- Aim for saturations of 94–98 per cent. If at risk of hypercarbia use target range of 88–92 per cent.		
Send bloods including cultures (glucose, lactate, FBC, U&Es, CRP, and Clotting). May need to consider lumbar puncture/other samples as indicated.		
Give IV antibiotics and consider source control. Maximum dose broad spectrum therapy. Refer to local policy, allergies, and antivirals.		
Give IV fluids Give up to 20 ml/kg fluid in divided boluses. Seek advice and give more fluid if indicated. Use lactate to help guide further fluid therapy.		
Monitor Use NEWS2. Measure and record urine output. May need to insert urinary catheter. Repeat lactate at least hourly if initial lactate elevated or clinical condition changes.		

Activity 6.3   Research

Please review the WHO surgical checklist. Please list the difference between this checklist and a care bundle.

An outline answer given at the end of this chapter.

Activity 6.4   Research

Please read around one of the following topics.

1. Care bundle – a five-step model for pressure ulcer prevention.
2. Sepsis 6 – a set of six tasks to be instituted within one hour by non-specialist practitioners at the frontline.
3. Intravenous device care bundle – includes central venous access devices (CVC) and peripheral access devices (PVC).
4. Alternatively, you may be aware of a care bundle that is used in your clinical area.

Make some notes and record the following.

- What are the different steps of the bundle?
- What is the evidence to support the different steps of the bundle?
- How is this information disseminated to teams?

As this activity is broad, there is no outline answer at the end of the chapter.

Challenges to care bundles

There may be a lack of compliance when introducing a care bundle and this can inhibit the successful implementation of a care bundle. Therefore, there needs to be staff education as this will improve staff engagement and motivation as well as appropriate resources. Some care bundles can appear overly complicated, and evidence suggests that the most successful care bundles are those with the least number of interventions (Gilhooly et al., 2019). There needs to be robust evidence to support each of the steps in a care bundle otherwise there is a risk of non-compliance in the implementation. There is a need for local or national regulation, otherwise there is a risk that anyone or a group of people can write a care bundle.

Care pathways

In contrast, a care pathway looks at the whole of a person's care from referral to investigation to treatment and will include the wider health and social care team. A care pathway is a complex process that involves decision-making across organisations to provide care for a well-defined group of people (Vanhaecht, 2007). The development of a care pathway may help to reduce health inequalities by ensuring people awaiting diagnosis or those with a diagnosis have access to evidence-based care in a timely manner. Organisations could measure their performance against agreed care pathways and use these data to either look at alternate ways of working or inject more funding to achieve specific outcomes. Getting it right first time (GIRFT) (see Table 6.7) are examples of care pathways such as the Paediatric acute abdominal pain and appendicectomy that sets out the best practice for managing a child who presents with acute abdominal pain (National Health Service, 2022).

Table 6.7   Getting it Right First Time

Presentation	Assessment and diagnosis	Pre/peri-operative care	Post-operative care
Presentation and initial assessment as per appendix pathway	Possible non-appendix cause of abdominal pain **Yes** – Perform appropriate investigations (e.g., blood tests, imaging) Surgical disease – **Yes** **No** – indication of surgical disease, consider non – surgical cause and discharge	Surgical disease indicated **Yes** – Clinical management: consider IV analgesia, IV fluids, and IV antibiotics Procedure or surgical intervention **Yes** – procedure or surgery undertaken **No** – clinical management plan as above, clinical review	Discharge when eating, drinking, pain controlled, afebrile, and fit for discharge

Activity 6.5   Research

Please research a care pathway that is relevant to your area of practice. If you are unsure, please ask your supervisor/team leader. Answer the following questions:

1.   Explain the client group for this care pathway.
2.   What are the pathway recommendations?
3.   What is the evidence-base?
4.   Is there a specified timeline for each step of the pathway? If so, what is it?
5.   Which professionals may be involved in the delivery of the care pathway?

There is no outline answer given at the end of this chapter.

Advantages of care pathways

Care pathways will lead to:

- enhanced communication between health and social care professionals, with patients and their families or carers;
- coordination of roles and sequencing of activities of the multidisciplinary care team, the patients and their families;
- improved documentation, monitoring of care and evaluating outcomes;
- identification of appropriate resources required.

Activity 6.6   Critical thinking

You have read about care pathways and understand the advantages of care pathways in practice. But what are the potential disadvantages of care pathways?

An outline answer is given at the end of this chapter.

Chapter summary

This chapter has introduced you to the principles of the nursing process and theories of nursing models. The case studies presented in this chapter will help to provide some context to help you understand the theories and apply to your clinical practice. Your role as an SNA/RNA has been described when considering the ongoing assessment, planning, implementation, review, and evaluation of nursing care. You have been introduced to models of care such as care bundles and care pathways that ensure care provided is evidence based. There will be a number of themes covered in this chapter that will be discussed elsewhere in this book.

Activities: Brief outline answers

Activity 6.1 Critical thinking (page 94)

There are five influencing factors from the Human Needs model and all factors will contribute to the planning and monitoring of patient care in the following ways.

Biological – Is the patient waiting any investigations, what is their medical history, how is that being managed, either pharmacologically or non-pharmacologically? Is there any deterioration?

Psychological – How is the person adapting to any illness, what are their coping strategies? Are they receiving any psychological support?

Sociocultural – Understanding a person's social circumstances can influence your care. For example, at a home visit you may notice that there is a cupboard full of medication, and it appears as though the person may not be taking prescribed medication. So, what do you need to consider now? Is a lack of concordance in taking medication causing symptoms?

Environmental – Understanding a person's environment can also influence your care. What are the person's beliefs about their environment? How are they contributing to the environment?

Political – Is the person able to influence their own changes? Do they understand local policies that may influence their care? Do they know how to access services? Who do they need to speak with?

Activity 6.2 Research (page 98)

Table 6.8   Activity 6.2 Suggested answer

Model	Views of the person	Goal of nursing	Knowledge and skills of the nurse
Family-centred care model	The child is a unique entity: a developing human being who has rights in law. The child is functioning, growing and developing, physically, emotionally, socially, intellectually, and spiritually.	Recognises that the goal of nursing is to support the parents or family members when caring for a child.	To understand the five aspects of nursing in child health that are the child, family, health, environment, and the nurse.
Tidal model	An individual's mental well-being is dependent on his or her individual life experiences, including his or her sense of self, perceptions, thoughts and actions.	Help individuals to create their own voyage of discovery.	The nurse uses a specific form of inquiry to explore the story collaboratively, revealing its hidden meanings, the patient's resources, and to identify what needs to be done to help the patient recover.

Activity 6.3 Research (page 100)

Table 6.9 Activity 6.3 Suggested answer

Care Bundle	WHO surgical checklist
Four or five interventions only listed	More interventions or steps
Box to confirm that the intervention or step has been completed or not	Box to confirm that the intervention or step has been completed or not
	Some not evidence-based but demonstrate good practice (e.g., Is the pulse oximeter on the patient and functioning?)
	Some interventions are evidence-based (e.g., the use of antibiotic prophylaxis)

Activity 6.6 Critical thinking (page 102)

The potential disadvantage of care pathways are as follows.

1. A reluctance among organisations and professionals to change, this reluctance may threaten the successful implementation of care pathways.
2. There may be difficulties engaging with care providers or clarifying people's roles and responsibilities. This can lead to variability in the implementation of care pathways.
3. It may not be clear to organisations and key stake holders whether integrated care influences patient outcomes.
4. Dehumanisation of work and a lack of creativity in the workplace.
5. The relationship between the health professional and the patient is less personal, due to a reduction in patient choice and less time for patient interaction.

Further reading

Royal College of Paediatrics and child health – Allergy Care Pathways. Available at:

www.rcpch.ac.uk/resources/clinical-guidelines-evidence-reviews/allergy-care-pathways.

A range of care pathways on paediatric and child health that relate to allergies such as allergy due to asthma and/or rhinitis, eczema, food and latex allergy.

Getting it right first time – Acute abdominal pain and appendicectomy pathway. Available at:

https://gettingitrightfirsttime.co.uk/wp-content/uploads/2022/06/20220607_Paediatric-general-surgery_Pathway-guide_Acute-abdominal-pain-and-appendicectomy.pdf.

The guide sets out a best practice pathway for managing paediatric acute abdominal pain and appendicectomy and to support improved outcomes for children in need of this service, and a sustainable NHS.

Getting it right first time – Paediatric forearm fracture manipulation pathway. Available at:

https://gettingitrightfirsttime.cc.uk/wp-content/uploads/2023/04/Paediatric-forearm-fracture-manipulation-pathway-FINAL-V1-April-2023.pdf.

This pathway supports hospital clinicians in treating children who present in the emergency department (ED) with a forearm fracture.

NHS Acute inpatient mental health care for adults and older adults. Available at:

www.england.nhs.uk/long-read/acute-inpatient-mental-health-care-for-adults-and-older-adults/

In 2019, the NHS Long Term Plan and NHS Mental Health Implementation Plan were published and set out an ambitious plan to transform mental health services. Unfortunately, shortly after publication, the COVID-19 pandemic began and this has had a major impact across the healthcare system, including mental health services. As a result of pandemic pressures and the increases in cost of living currently facing households, inpatient mental health services have experienced sustained rises in demand and acuity, which have been particularly challenging due to the current workforce pressures across the NHS. This guidance aims to support the commissioning and delivery of high-quality inpatient care, close to home and in the least restrictive way.

Achieving better access to 24/7 urgent and emergency mental health care. Available at:

www.england.nhs.uk/publication/achieving-better-access-to-247-urgent-and-emergency-mental-health-care-part-2-implementing-the-evidence-based-treatment-pathway-for-urgent-and-emergency-liaison-mental-health-services-for/

This guide is part of a series for urgent and emergency mental health care that also covers 'blue light' services (for all ages), community-based crisis response services (for adults and older adults) and children and young people's crisis services.

National Partnership Agreement: Right Care, Right Person (RCRP). Available at:

www.gov.uk/government/publications/national-partnership-agreement-right-care-right-person/national-partnership-agreement-right-care-right-person-rcrp

The Right Care, Right Person' (RCRP) provides a framework for assisting police with decision-making about when they should be involved in responding to reported incidents involving people with mental health needs.

Useful websites

www.longtermplan.nhs.uk/about/

The NHS Long Term plan was published in 2019 and agreed to a commitment to improve and secure funding for the NHS; recognised the need for change and that this needed to include service users, family, carers as well as healthcare professionals; and provide practical experiences of changes that have happened.

www.ndti.org.uk/assets/files/The_Health_Equality_Framework_final_word.pdf

The Health Equalities Framework (HEF), an outcomes framework based on the determinants of health inequalities. This document provides guidance on the HEF structure, as well instructions on how to rate the presenting circumstances of a person with a learning disability.

https://nandadiagnosis.com

A nursing diagnosis is an essential component of nursing practice that helps nurses identify actual or potential health problems. NANDA (North American Nursing Diagnosis Association) is the principal organisation for defining standardised nursing diagnosis. This webpage provides a list of nursing diagnosis.

www.rcpch.ac.uk/

Royal College of Paediatrics and Child Health.

The Royal College of Paediatrics and Child Health is an international membership body for paediatricians. The group provide professional standards, further education, professional standards, policy and further research. The website provides a useful section on resources and key topics.

www.who.int/teams/integrated-health-services/patient-safety/research/safe-surgery/tool-and-resources

The WHO Surgical Safety checklist was developed to promote safety, increase teamwork and communication in surgery. This webpage provides additional information about safe surgery.

Consider the wider determinants of health when providing and monitoring care

Hazel Cowls and Sarah Tobin

NMC *STANDARDS FOR PROFICIENCY FOR NURSING ASSOCIATES*

This chapter will address the following platforms and proficiencies.

Platform 1: Being an accountable practitioner

1.1   understand and act in accordance with the Code: Professional standards of practice and behaviour for nurses, midwives and nursing associates and fulfil all registration requirements.

Platform 2: Promoting health and preventing ill health

2.4   understand the factors that may lead to inequalities in health outcomes.

Platform 3: Provide and monitor care

Annexe A: Communication and relationship management skills

4. Demonstrate effective communication skills for working in professional teams.

Chapter aims

After reading this chapter, you will be able to:

- demonstrate an understanding of wider determinants of health;
- explore the impact of wider/social determinants on health outcomes for individuals and communities;
- review how health inequalities are being managed at a national and local level.

Introduction

In Chapter 2, you were introduced to the idea of health inequalities and how there are wider determinants that impact a person's health and well-being. In Chapter 3, you explored how the biopsychosocial model is a holistic approach that enables healthcare professionals to consider an individual's social circumstances and all aspects of their physical and mental well-being. In this chapter, you are going to build on this knowledge by exploring the impact of wider determinants of health, such as income, education and environmental factors, when providing and monitoring patient care. As with many aspects of nursing and care provision as a whole, the concept of wider determinants is really common sense – someone who cannot read or does not have easy access to transport or has a limited income will face more challenges than a person who does not face these restrictions. However, even though it may seem like common sense to acknowledge this, evidence highlights that policy, infrastructure and training (as just some examples) does not adequately address this need. Put simply – accessing the healthcare that people need is significantly impacted by a number of different social, economic, environmental, and structural factors. These need to be acknowledged and addressed, at a national level, but also at every level of service provision including when assessing the patient sat in front of you.

The Nursing Associate Curriculum Framework (HEE, 2017) which underpinned the initial education programmes for RNAs highlighted that it is a requirement to demonstrate knowledge and understanding of 'socioeconomic factors and wider determinants of health'. This underlines the importance placed on this as a major factor when caring for patients; additionally, the document stated the need to 'reflect on the role of the nursing associate in taking these factors into account in the delivery of care and supporting the planning of care'.

So, what are the 'wider determinants of health'?

According to the Office for Health Improvement and Disparities (2022):

> Wider determinants, also known as social determinants, are a diverse range of social, economic and environmental factors which impact on people's health. Such factors are influenced by the local, national and international distribution of power and resources which shape the conditions of daily life.

This is a very neat explanation of what is a very complex set of circumstances but boils down to the key concepts of resource and power. Information is a very significant resource and a powerful tool, and health education has been a key issue in addressing wider determinants.

Activity 7.1   Review and reflect

In Chapter 2, you were asked to list the seven factors that combine to form the index of deprivation and also identify the groups of people who will be more vulnerable to health inequalities. Return to Activity 2.4 and either research for these answers or look at the model answer at the end of Chapter 2.

Take some time to consider how all of these factors can impact on a person's health and well-being – not simply their physical health but their mental health and their sense of security as well as opportunity and even hope.

If we agree that health is, as the WHO (1946) suggests, 'a state of complete physical, mental and social well-being and not merely the absence of disease or infirmity' then it becomes clearer how these elements can and do impact on an individual's health.

As this is a reflective exercise no model answer is provided but...read on for further information and context, so keep the reflection going.

These factors are very impactful when assessing a person's needs and planning their care and this holds true for an individual person or an entire population. The important thing to remember is that health inequalities are both unfair and, generally, avoidable differences between disparate groups of people in society. Health service planners therefore have an obligation to try to 'level up' (a much-used political concept in recent years in the United Kingdom) the care provided to address the lack of fairness and access. And, before you read on...remember that these wider determinants can literally impact how long a person might live or how healthy they will be while they live, it really is that important.

The conditions into which we are born, where we grow up, work, play and age are all important factors and are often interlinked. It's not surprising that a person who is unemployed is likely to live in poorer housing, have less access to leisure activities and will perhaps even eat a less healthy diet. If these circumstances persist then, inevitably, the risk of poorer health increases while the access to health services is more challenging.

The reasons for the link between poorer health and wider determinants are complex; NHS England (2022) suggests that the following may be some of the reasons:

- the availability of services in their local area;
- service opening times;
- access to transport;
- access to childcare;
- language (spoken and written);
- literacy;
- poor experiences in the past;
- misinformation;
- fear.

People who experience perhaps just one of these challenges may be able to manage, but often those who experience inequalities find the challenges are compounded – one problem leading to another. So, if you have no-one to look after your children, a limited income and the bus stop is a mile away with infrequent buses, how easy is it to attend the breast screening appointment you have been sent?

It is also important to consider that those living in areas of high deprivation who are from 'inclusion health groups' are at even greater disadvantage and therefore risk According to NHS England, inclusion health is an umbrella term used to describe people who are socially excluded, who typically experience multiple overlapping risk factors for poor health, such as poverty, violence and complex trauma. This includes people who experience homelessness, drug and alcohol dependence, vulnerable migrants, Gypsy, Roma and Traveller communities, sex workers, people in contact with the justice system and victims of modern slavery.

Case study 7.1: Jenny

You are an RNA working in a community health centre, one of the remits of the centre is to provide outreach support to a local homeless shelter and to the wider community of homeless people. Jenny is approximately 45 years old; she sporadically accesses the homeless shelter for hot food and to use the washing facilities that they provide. Jenny is not very willing to engage with staff, keeps herself to herself and usually refuses much in the way of the help or interventions offered. From what little is known, it appears that Jenny has experienced domestic abuse and subsequently became home-less. Her mental health is concerning as staff state that Jenny has seemed confused at times and often appears to have been drinking alcohol to excess. Her appearance can be unkempt, but staff note that Jenny tries to keep herself as clean and well-presented as possible, the use of their washing facilities is one of the ways that they try to provide support.

Jenny arrives at the unit and, unusually, asks if she can see a nurse. You are in the Shelter and agree to see Jenny who asks you to come into the washroom with her – there she shows you an ulcerated, moist lesion on her left breast. The wound is approximately six centimetres across, foul smelling and clearly very sore as Jenny grimaces and shakes as she removes the tissue paper she has used to cover it. On gentle questioning Jenny tells you she noticed the start of the ulcer several months ago and has been trying to manage it herself, she is scared of doctors and hospital and hoped it would heal up on its own. It is now very painful, and she has, reluctantly, decided to ask for some help.

Activity 7.2   Skill

Consider how you might help Jenny and what wider determinants you will need to consider that will have to be addressed in any assessment and plan of care.

Some ideas and suggestions are included in a model answer at the end of the chapter.

A model to help understand wider determinants

Several models have been developed to help broaden people's understanding of the concept of health, moving beyond individual responsibility by looking at the root causes of ill health. The most widely used is the Dahlgren-Whitehead model first presented in 1991 and shown in Figure 7.1.

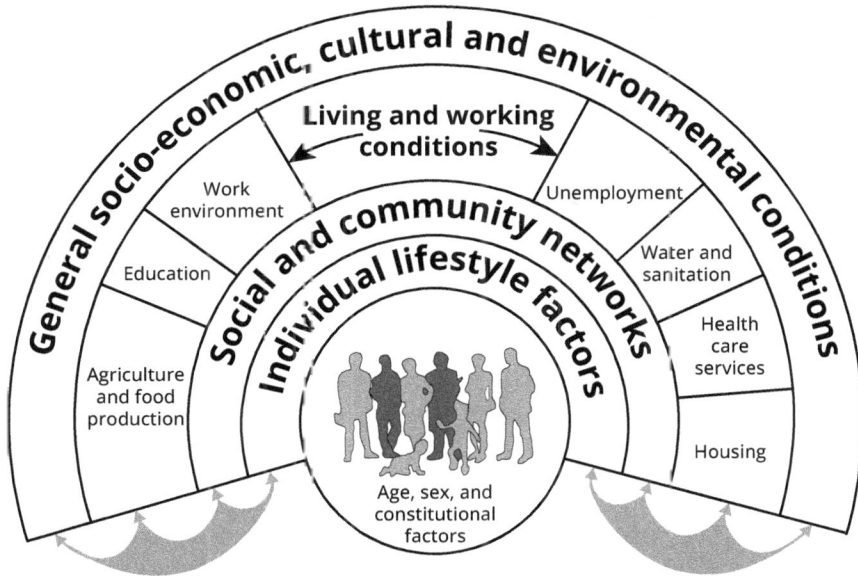

Figure 7.1   The main determinants of health

Source: adapted from Dahlgren and Whitehead, 1991.

The model is, understandably, known as the 'Rainbow model' and was created to *'visually illustrate the layers of influence on population health and provide a simple framework for thinking about the policy response of the different sectors involved in tackling these determinants'* (Dahlgren and Whitehead, 2021). The strength of the model according to the authors is that it takes a holistic view of the main determinants and is easy to follow. The elements of the rainbow can be health promoting, protective (e.g., vaccines) or health-damaging risks. Other models have been developed but these often focus mainly on risk factors – what to prevent rather than what to promote or the determinants of health rather than the causes of disease.

Thirty years after the model was developed, Dahlgren and Whitehead (2021) suggested that to reflect current healthcare the model needs to be adapted. They describe three areas that need consideration. First, the need to better demonstrate the link between the social, economic, and cultural determinants of health and lifestyle. This is because lifestyle is not simply a choice but is often shaped by the social and economic environment – for instance, choosing to eat or provide a healthy diet depends not only on choice but also on income and what food is accessible. The second area is the impact of commercial activity, specifically the strategies of food, alcohol, and tobacco companies used to promote their products. They also link this aspect to pollution, to access to health care, to access to education – almost all aspects of our lives are not determined by genetics. Finally, the authors describe a growing debate about the influence of racism on health and whether it should be incorporated as a determinant of health. They felt that the driving force of racism, including discrimination and institutional and structural racism, impacts on all the social, economic, cultural, and environmental conditions in society.

This model, as with all models, will need to be constantly adapted to reflect the changes in the societies in which we live.

What is the impact of wider/social determinants on health outcomes for individuals and communities?

The statistics illustrate notable variation in life expectancy from birth in UK countries, as shown below:

- England, 78.8 years for males and 82.8 years for females.
- Scotland, 76.5 years for males and 80.7 years for females.
- Wales, 77.9 years for males and 81.8 years for females.
- Northern Ireland, 78.4 years for males and 82.3 years for females (Office for National Statistics, 2024).

Looking more specifically at London Boroughs, for example in Kensington and Chelsea, the life expectancy at birth for males is 80.67 and for females is 86.34 compared to Barking some 14 miles away, where the life expectancy for male is 76.26 and for females is 80.44. So, what factors contribute to people dying prematurely? In 2010, the Marmot Review (Marmot et al., 2010) highlighted that in England, people were dying prematurely because of health inequalities. The review acknowledged that health inequalities arise because of unfair conditions within society such as where people are born, grow, live, work, and age, recognising that the lower a person's socio-economic position the worse their health. For example, children who have a low cognitive score at 22 months of age but who grow up in families with a higher socio-economic position will improve their cognitive score as they approach 10 years of age. In contrast, children with a high cognitive score at 22 months of age but who grow up in families with a lower socio-economic position will have a worse score as they approach 10 years of age.

Furthermore, there is evidence that rates of unemployment in adulthood are associated with an increased risk of mortality and morbidity due to:

- limiting long-term illness;
- cardiovascular disease;
- poor mental health;
- suicidal ideation;
- health-harming behaviours.

The impact of unemployment and ill-health also affects families and the economy. In 2018, in the United Kingdom (UK) there were an estimated 32.4 million people in work and the employment rate for people aged 16–64 years was 75.7 per cent. However, there were 1.38 million people unemployed; that is, people not in work but seeking employment with an estimated rate of unemployment of 4.1 per cent. A further 8.74 million people (aged 16–64 years) were economically inactive, unemployed and not seeking employment with an estimated rate of economic inactivity at 21.2 per cent. It is recognised that 1 in 6 employees in the United Kingdom have reported experiencing a mental health condition such as stress, anxiety and depression leading to sick absence. There is a substantial employment rate gap in the United Kingdom between disabled and non-disabled people, with only 51.3 per cent of disabled people being in employment. The *Health Matters: health and work* document (Public Health England, 2019) aims to protect against social exclusion due to low income, social interaction, a person's identity and recognises that good work is important.

The Marmot Review (2010) suggested the following actions to promote fairness and reduce inequalities:

1. Ensure every child has the best start in life.
2. Enable all children young people and adults to maximise their capabilities and have control over their lives.
3. Create fair employment and good work for everyone.
4. Ensure a healthy standard of living for everyone.
5. Create and develop healthy and sustainable places and communities.
6. Strengthen the role and impact of ill health prevention.

An update of the original 2010 Marmot Review, *Health Equity in England: The Marmot Review 10 Years On* (Marmot et al., 2020) highlighted that health inequalities, rather than improving, have been increasing and, for the whole population, health is declining. The report summarised by stating actions were required in all six recommendations above. So, what can be done about this? The Office for Health Improvements and Disparities (OHID) is part of the Department of Health and Social Care. The OHID focuses on improving the health of the nation so that everyone can expect to live in good health, and on levelling up health disparities or inequalities to break down the link between a person's background and prospects for living a healthy life. Later in this chapter, you will explore actions that aim to reduce health inequalities.

As an SNA or RNA, you need to understand how the social determinants of health will impact a person's health and well-being and, working with individuals, identify how these can be managed.

Next, we introduce you to Avery and Luca who have both accessed health services. As you are reading the case studies make a note of the social determinants that may impact each person's health.

Case study 7.2: Avery

The community nursing team received a referral from a local GP to obtain a blood sample for routine screening prior to commencing antipsychotic medication. Limited information on the referral form. Avery aged 62 years old, previously long-term resident at a local hospital that cared for people with mental health illness. Avery resided at the hospital for over 30 years. The community nursing team lead requested that the RNA visits Avery to collect a blood sample.

First visit by RNA – Avery would only open the door and would not let the RNA enter the property. The RNA spoke calmly and explained the need to enter the property to take a blood sample prior to commencing the medication as prescribed by the doctor. Avery agreed that the RNA could return the following day to take a blood sample.

Second visit by RNA – The RNA was able to enter the property. The RNA noticed that Avery was hoarding as there were items everywhere, down the stairs, in the hallway. Avery stated that *'during the "lockdown" of 2020, I stayed in my home. I did not go outside at all, and I don't go outside now. I request food deliveries online and they leave my food at the door. I wait for them to leave before I open the door. I do not have any family and no friends to speak to, so I just stay indoors. I feel safer here anyway'*.

During the home visit the RNA noticed that Avery had dressings on both legs and on further inspection he had bilateral leg ulcers that required treatment. The RNA arranged with Avery, and the team leader, to visit Avery three times a week initially to commence treatment.

(Continued)

Subsequent visits by RNA – The RNA recognised that Avery appeared scared and was fearful of going outside. Avery did not like meeting new people, but the RNA did introduce Avery to another member of the team to ensure that care could be continuous if the RNA was not available.

In the first case study, we meet Avery who lives alone and has become isolated preferring to remain indoors, initially to reduce the transference of the SARS-CoV-2 pathogen, ordering online shopping to limit contact with people. Unfortunately, this practice has led to Avery not seeking healthcare advise when he developed leg ulcers and it appears on inspection that he has been trying to manage the treatment himself. It is possible that Avery needs to rebuild trust with the nursing associate and others. As an SNA or RNA, you need to be respectful of the choices made by a person, taking time to build trust. In this case the RNA recognised that Avery did not like meeting new people, but the RNA needed to ensure continuing care so introduced Avery to a colleague.

The Office for National Statistics (ONS, 2023) stated that approximately 8.4 million people in the United Kingdom were living alone. There has been a significant increase in people living alone in older age groups (65 years). There is a variation in life expectancy between the sexes, with women typically living longer than men and this creates more one person households among the older population. If we look at other age groups, those aged 25–64, it is mainly men who live alone (60 per cent) but the gap between the sexes narrows as we age. These statistics matter as the Health Foundation (2018) stated that living alone increases the risk of social isolation and loneliness and that a lack of social connection has proven harmful to health comparable to smoking 15 cigarettes a day.

In relation to Avery's case and other people in similar circumstances an RNA stated that:

'As an RNA working in the community, it was common practice for me to speak to patients about hygiene and wound care'.

Case study 7.3: Luca

Luca, aged 48 years, has been suffering with poor mental health for many years and is supported by the community mental health team. They also have been diagnosed with diabetes, myocardial infarction and new terminology. Heart Failure with Reduced Ejection Fraction (HFrEF). They attend the GP clinic for management of cardiovascular disease. Unfortunately, Luca has not been coping well at home and is admitted to hospital with decompensated heart failure. You are the RNA allocated to care for Luca and are interested in finding out about their social circumstances, as this forms part of their assessment and will aid discharge planning. Luca informs you that they have an older brother who lives approximately 200 miles away and a niece, but he does not see them very much. Luca lives in shared housing, explaining that they have their own room but share communal kitchen, living area and laundry. Luca enjoys reading and has previously joined a reading group but has not attended the group for a while. They are unemployed and receive benefits from the government *'but that does not go very far'*. This is Luca's story.

'The doctor prescribed a water tablet; I think it is called a diuretic. I know I must go to the toilet frequently in the morning, but I can't move very well, so sometimes I have an accident, you know pass urine and soil my trousers. I don't like using the washing machine as other people use it, and I worry that people will know I have had an accident. I feel so embarrassed. What do I do? Well, I just throw my trousers away. Yes, it does get expensive. I cannot afford a new pair of trousers; money doesn't go very far nowadays. I thought it may help if I stopped taking the water tablet, you know the diuretic. But it hasn't really, my legs are so swollen, I cannot move very well. I am retaining fluid, and I think that is why I am in hospital.'

This case study illustrates the importance of listening to people to find out about the real issue that people are facing and working together to find a solution. As an RNA or SNA, what else can you do to help Luca? From the case study, you may have identified a few areas of concern. Firstly, does Luca have a good understanding of his condition and does he know how to manage his symptoms effectively? Luca reported that he had not been 'coping well at home', so do you need to speak with Luca about a referral to physiotherapy and occupational therapy? Luca may be experiencing financial worries, so is he eligible for any financial support and who is available to help Luca ensure he has access to all support? Luca's family live far away, so do they have any other people around who can help if required? Luca may benefit from meeting a social prescriber as they can signpost Luca to organisations and groups that may be of interest to Luca.

Poor mental health, as in Luca's case, may have an impact on a person's quality of life (Department of Health, 2011) and their life expectancy, with people living 15–20 years less than the general population (Public Health England [PHE], 2018) that is largely due to physical ill-health (OHID, 2023). For example, the mortality rate for people with severe mental health compared to the general population is:

- 3.3 times higher for cardiovascular disease;
- 2 times higher for cancer;
- 5 times higher for liver disease;
- 4.7 times higher for respiratory disease (PHE, 2018).

Working in partnership with the person involved and all agencies such as community services and social prescribing will lead to an effective, safe discharge and reduce the occurrence of readmission. The hospital discharge and community support guidance provide statutory guidelines to NHS bodies that include NHS Trusts, integrated care boards (ICBs) and local authorities (Department of Health and Social Care, 2024).

Activity 7.3 Research

Review local hospital policy on hospital discharge and community support guidelines. Are there any other community organisations that can support people on discharge from hospital?

As this activity is based on your own observation, there is no outline answer at the end of the chapter.

Activity 7.4   Critical thinking

Social Prescribing is a key component of personalised care, and NHS England is committed to building an infrastructure for social prescribing across the NHS. Please review the National Academy for Social Prescribing (NASP) available online at: https://socialprescribingacademy.org.uk/

As this activity is based on your own observation, there is no outline answer at the end of the chapter.

The wider costs of health inequalities

In 2022, the Department for Work and Pensions conducted a review and analysed different data streams to assess the overall financial implications of ill health to the United Kingdom. The estimated cost to the economy was based on:

- lost production because of economic inactivity due to long-term or temporary sickness;
- lost production due to sickness absence;
- lost production due to informal care giving which removes people from the workforce;
- additional costs to the NHS when someone's health condition causes them to move from economically active to economically inactive;
- lost Tax and forgone National Insurance returns to the Exchequer due to health conditions preventing or limiting employment;
- cost of social security benefits related to health conditions that prevent people from working.

The figures did not include the costs associated with working age mortality (a key social determinant) as robust enough data did not exist which would enable accurate assessment.

A caring society should always make provision for those who through no fault of their own are unable to work, to support those who are ill. However, if that number is increased by preventable health inequalities, then the cost to society will be unnecessarily increased – not just in terms of unnecessary suffering but also in an increased financial burden. Even without the data from premature deaths, the cost of supporting working age people who are sick, or disabled is approximately £259 billion, a figure that almost doubled from the previous review in 2016.

Imagine if even a modest reduction in sickness levels could be achieved by reducing the impact of health inequalities and wider determinants. The benefits would not just be in healthier people but also, in some circumstances, in people who may no longer need financial support and could be productive workers who contribute to the economy – a double benefit.

How health inequalities are being managed at a national and local level: CORE20PLUS5

NHS England is committed to reducing healthcare inequalities at both national and systems level. The Core20PLUS5 programme is in three parts. Part one focuses on 'Core20' that refers to the most deprived 20 per cent of the national population as identified by the

Index of Multiple Deprivation (IMD; NHS England, 2019). The IMD is the official measure of deprivation in England and is based on numerous factors in a person's life such as finances as well as access to resources. The seven domains of deprivation are listed below in Table 7.1.

Understanding the theory

Table 7.1 The seven domains of deprivation combined create the IMD

Income	Employment	Education	Health	Crime	Barriers to housing	Living environment
22.5 per cent	22.5 per cent	13.5 per cent	13.5 per cent	9.3 per cent	9. per cent	9.3 per cent
Proportion of people on low income.	Proportion of people, working age involuntarily excluded from the labour market.	Measures the lack of attainment and skills in the local population.	Measures the risk of premature death and the impairment of quality of life through poor physical or mental health.	Measures the risk of personal and material victimisation at a local level.	Measures the physical and financial accessibility of housing and local services.	Measures the quality of the indoor and outdoor local environment.

Part two 'PLUS' refers to population groups such as ethnic minority communities; inclusion health groups (people experiencing homelessness, drug and alcohol dependence, vulnerable migrants, Traveller communities, sex workers, people known to criminal justice system and victims of modern slavery); people with a learning disability and autistic people to name a few.

Part three '5' refers to the five areas that require accelerated improvement and these are different for adults and children as listed below:

Adult areas:

- maternity services;
- severe mental illness;
- chronic respiratory disease;
- early cancer diagnosis;
- hypertension case-finding and optimal management and lipid optimal management.

Children's areas:

- asthma;
- diabetes;
- epilepsy;
- oral health;
- mental health.

The projects below are some examples of best practice to reduce health inequalities.

Project 1. The aim of the project was to reduce significant differences in hypertension management at two GP practices. At the start of the project, 67 per cent of white and only 55 per cent of black patients aged under 80 with hypertension were being treated to target, representing a 12 per cent inequality gap. The project ran for one year and involved a few health care professionals contacting patients registered at the practice to provide guidance and education around self-care, and information about lifestyle approaches and medication. The results of the project showed that with the intervention 87 per cent of all patients aged under 80 with hypertension are now well controlled.

Project 2. A city centre clinic that provides support to people experiencing homelessness, insecure housing, refugees and asylum seekers, and vulnerable women. The street health bus provides an outreach clinic to people who may not usually access health services.

Read more about how people and organisations have been looking to reduce health inequalities at the NHS Equality and Health Inequalities Hub. Available online at: www.england.nhs.uk/about/equality/equality-hub/case-studies/

Activity 7.5   Research

Are you aware of what is happening in your community to reduce healthcare inequalities? Choose a population group (e.g., PLUS such as ethnic minority group, travelling community, someone who is dependent on drugs or alcohol) and then choose one of the five areas that require accelerated improvements. Make a note of the following:

1.   What is the improvement?
2.   Who is involved?
3.   How is this information shared with people in the community?
4.   How will we know if this has been successful?

As this activity is based on your own observation, there is no outline answer at the end of the chapter.

Health inequalities - not just an urban problem

The problems of inner cities have been widely documented. Housing stock in some areas may typically be old and in poor condition, especially where housing was associated with industries that have closed down or where social changes altered housing – the move to high-rise buildings in the 1960s for instance. High density populations require high levels of employment and when an area can no longer provide enough jobs the whole community becomes affected. So-called urban decay has been the subject of a great deal of policy initiatives and some funding streams for social improvement.

High populations also bring increased amounts of traffic and therefore an increase in pollution levels. Several recent high-profile cases have highlighted this. Ella Adoo-Kissi-Debrah who lived near the south circular road in Lewisham, South-East London died in 2013 aged just nine years. Ella died as a result of an asthma attack but an inquest in 2020 found that air pollution made a material contribution to her death. Ella was the first person in the United Kingdom to have air pollution listed as a cause of death which the government's own adviser called 'a landmark decision' (BBC, 2020). And in 2022 an inquest found that the death of two-year-old Awaab Ishak was due to respiratory disease caused by exposure to environmental mould – the little boy lived in social housing that was not fit for human habitation. Awaab's family had arrived from Sudan as refugees before he was born, his father repeatedly raised concerns about the state of their home, but no action was taken. Subsequent investigations discovered other houses on the same estate were in equally bad if not worse condition.

It is clear that poor housing and pollution can significantly impact a person's health, with the potential for tragic consequences. So, it would be easy to assume that living in the countryside would be much more beneficial and the risk of health inequalities also less impactful. However, while there are definite benefits of rural living there are also significant challenges. The fact that when Public Health England was disbanded in 2021, the new organisation that took over public health responsibilities was called the Office for Health Improvement and **Disparities** suggests that not everything in the garden is rosy! As an example, one of the most popular holiday destinations in the United Kingdom with over five million annual visitors is the undeniably beautiful county of Cornwall. However, just before the COVID-19 pandemic (after which a lot of data was impacted and 'skewed') Cornwall was identified as the second poorest region in the whole of Northern Europe (second only to West Wales....also in the United Kingdom) according to figures produced by Eurostat, the data agency of the European Union. In fact, 9 of the top 10 of the poorest areas were from the United Kingdom and many were predominantly rural in nature (although the richest region was also in the United Kingdom – London – clearly highlighting the lack of equality in the United Kingdom).

Activity 7.6   Critical thinking

Considering all that you have read about the wider determinants of health and resultant health inequalities make a list of all of the factors that could impact on the health challenges of the population of Cornwall.

A model answer has been provided at the end of the chapter.

Conclusion

The privilege of good health is a precious, our most precious, asset – as individuals and within our communities and wider society. Being healthy enables us to lead happy and fulfilling lives – health underpins our ability to achieve our potential, to feel a sense of worth and achievement and to enable positive social and economic outcomes. The health of a nation is its foundation – healthy children grow and thrive and reach their educational potential, a healthy workforce is productive and supports a nation's economy. Healthy people are happier, have a better income, more choices, more opportunity and live longer and more independently. Aneurin Bevan (1897–1960) who spearheaded the establishment of the NHS in 1947 said, 'No society can legitimately call itself civilized if a sick person is denied medical aid because of lack of means'. In the 1940s this statement related to the fact that healthcare was not free and only those with enough money could access medical care. However, the concept of access remains as relevant and as impactful now as it did then – wider determinants and health inequality – 'lack of means' – result in lack of access to 'medical aid' just as surely now as then.

In order to ensure nurses stay at the forefront of civilised society, we need to be educated about the inequalities some of our patients face. The Standards of Proficiency for Nursing Associates (2024) make this clear, within Platform 2, 2.3 states that RNAs need to be able to describe the principles of demography and the influence this has on health and well-being. 2.4 states the RNA needs to understand the factors that may lead to inequalities in health outcomes and 2.6 highlights the importance of social influences, health literacy, individual circumstances, behaviours and lifestyle choices on mental, physical, and behavioural health outcomes. This knowledge needs to underpin your nursing assessments to ensure that they respond to the individual and the challenges they may face. Without such informed and personalised assessment no plan of care will provide fair and equal access to care for patients.

Chapter summary

This chapter has introduced you to the concepts of the wider determinants of health and how health care can be unequal in access and provision. A widely adopted model (Dahlgren and Whitehead, 1991) has been described which can be used as a visual cue to broaden understanding of health and what impacts and supports good health. The impact to health and the economic costs of the wider determinants and inequalities has been described as have some initiatives to address inequality both locally and nationally. The fact that health inequalities are not confined to one area or environment is explored as well as the implications of this. Throughout the chapter the importance of an individual's ability to access health and well-being services is linked to the need for individualised assessment and care planning.

Activities - brief outline answers:

Activity 7.2 (page 110)

The most important factor that will determine the help you might provide is Jenny herself. The most important consideration will be an assessment of Jenny's priorities and wishes as assessment will drive the subsequent plan of care and needs to be mutually agreed. In Jenny's situation it will be necessary to ensure that her view and not that of the care staff is established – this will be especially difficult as a likely cause of the lesion Jenny shows the RNA is that of a malignancy. It may be that Jenny will not accept invasive investigations or treatment, that a formal diagnosis is not her priority – whatever her view and however unwise, as long as she has capacity this will need to be respected (see the Mental Capacity Act 2005 for more information). So, the first thing is to establish her views, her wishes and her priorities – and to document these clearly.

The wider determinants that will need to be considered include:

- Her living conditions – where does she sleep, find shelter/warmth/food.
- Her social support network – any input of family or friends.
- Her financial situation.
- Her access to health education and information.
- Her underlying dependence on alcohol or other substances.
- Any other underlying health conditions not yet identified or treated.
- How she will access support in future, especially if not local.

Activity 7.5 Critical thinking (page 119)

Some of the issues that impact on health inequalities in Cornwall include:

- Average income – in Cornwall this is around 80 per cent of the national average.
- Lack of permanent employment opportunity, high rates of seasonal employment.
- High incidence of families and children living in poverty.
- High rates of homelessness
- Poor transport links (poor access to services – health, education) so high transport costs.
- A rural and spread-out population (increased risk of isolation).
- High housing costs (large gap between the most affluent and the poorest pushes up housing costs).
- Loss of European Union funding (Cornwall received more economic aid from the EU than any other part of the United Kingdom).
- Poor or old housing stock – e.g., almost half the county does not have access to mains gas (14 per cent do not nationally), increased fuel poverty.

Further reading and useful websites

Fair society, healthy lives: the Marmot Review: strategic review of health inequalities in England post-2010. Available at: www.gov.uk/research-for-development-outputs/fair-society-healthy-lives-the-marmot-review-strategic-review-of-health-inequalities-in-england-post-2010

This review looks at the most effective ways to reduce health inequalities.

Health Equity in England: The Marmot Review 10 Years On. Available at: www.health.org.uk/publications/reports/the-marmot-review-10-years-on

This report is ten years on from the Fair Society, Healthy Lives (Marmot Review) highlighting that people can expect to spend more of their lives in poor health; the health gap has grown between wealthy and deprived areas; improvements in life expectancy have stalled and declined for women in most deprived areas.

NHS England, National Health Inequalities Programme.

Core 20 plus 5 (adult) Available at: www.england.nhs.uk/about/equality/equality-hub/national-healthcare-inequalities-improvement-programme/core20plus5/

Core 20 plus 5 (children and young people) Available at: www.england.nhs.uk/about/equality/equality-hub/national-healthcare-inequalities-improvement-programme/core20plus5/core20plus5-cyp/

NHS England has launched the Core20PLUS5 to support the reduction of health inequalities at both national and system level. The approach will target specific population cohort and identifies '5' focus clinical areas requiring accelerated improvement.

Social Determinants of Health (World Health Organisation). Available at: www.who.int/health-topics/social-determinants-of-health#tab=tab_1 Further information on the social determinants of health throughout the world. Review key concepts of social determinants here.

NICE and health inequalities. Available at: www.nice.org.uk/about/what-we-do/nice-and-health-inequalities.

Explore how NICE can help tackle health inequalities.

The importance of sensitive and compassionate assessment and planning for all people

Sarah Tobin

NMC *STANDARDS OF PROFICIENCY FOR NURSING ASSOCIATES*

This Chapter will address the following platforms and proficiencies.

Platform 1: Being an accountable professional

1.1 understand and act in accordance with The Code: Professional standards of practice and behaviour for nurses, midwives and nursing associates, and fulfil all registration requirements.

Platform 1: Being an accountable practitioner

1.10 demonstrate the skills and abilities required to develop, manage and maintain appropriate relationships with people, their families, carers, and colleague.

Platform 3: Provide and monitor care

3.6 demonstrate the knowledge, skills and ability to perform a range of nursing procedures and manage devices, to meet people's need for safe and effective person-centred care.

3.13 demonstrate an understanding of how to deliver sensitive and compassionate end of life care to support people to plan for their end of life, giving information and support to people who are dying, their families and the bereaved. Provide care to the deceased.

Annex A

2.9 engage in difficult conversations with support from others, helping people who are feeling emotionally or physically vulnerable or in distress, conveying compassion and sensitivity.

Chapter aims

After reading this chapter you will be able to:

- Define compassion and demonstrate an understanding of how it underpins safe and effective care provision.
- Understand how assessment and planning that is based on compassionate principles can be delivered.
- Begin to explore the importance of compassionate cultures and how you as an individual professional can contribute and benefit from them.
- Develop an understanding of some of the unique (but transferrable) elements of the provision of compassionate and sensitive end of life care.

Introduction

The previous chapters in this book have emphasised the importance of planning individualised, holistic care for people based on adequate assessment of their biopsychosocial needs and considering the wider determinants that impact health and well-being. This final chapter will consider the impact of compassion as an underpinning, clinically impactful approach to assessing, planning, and evaluating care. The first sentence of the first Platform of the Standards of Proficiency for Nursing Associates (NMC, 2024) states: 'Nursing associates act in the best interests of people, putting them first and providing nursing care that is person-centred, safe and **compassionate**'. So, to provide compassion-based care is not simply a good and decent thing to do, it is a professional obligation, mandated by the SNA/RNAs regulatory body!

And, compassionate care is not just a nice concept, something that in the past may have been described as a 'soft skill'; an increasing body of evidence demonstrates that compassionate care has significant clinical impact. And, in a challenging and resource-poor healthcare environment, compassion has also proved a sustainable way to provide care. Finally, when healthcare professionals are facing significant levels of stress and burn-out, the provision of care with compassion acts as a protection for staff, supporting their well-being and reducing attrition.

So, what is compassion?

This may seem to be a strange question as I am sure you will already have an idea in your mind, your own definition of what compassion means and even what it looks like in practice.

Understanding the theory – why definition matters

The renowned clinical psychologist Paul Gilbert highlighted the need to understand a phenomenon by agreeing a set of properties unique to it. He used the example of a discussion about a chair, an elephant, a tiger and a cat – all share the quality of being four-legged things, but all are clearly very different. If a discussion, a policy or a guideline is to be meaningful then there will need to be an explicit and common understanding, or one person will be talking about a chair whilst their colleague is discussing a tiger! So, we need to be specific and clear about what we mean by the term 'compassion'. This is especially important as there are many words that seem to be used interchangeably, terms such as empathy, caring, kindness, humanity, and even civility.

A definition is an important requirement in a chapter that sets out to demonstrate the importance of compassion in providing effective care. The dictionary would have us know compassion as 'sympathetic consciousness of others' distress together with a desire to alleviate it' (Merriam-Webster, 2025). A simple definition may be helpful but is not focused or comprehensive enough to explain compassion in a healthcare context. Linguistically, the term 'compassion' is derived from the Latin root 'com', which means 'together with' and 'pati', which is 'to bear or suffer'. This definition – effectively to suffer with – is contentious in healthcare professions where the body of evidence to support the increasing level of 'burnout' and compassion fatigue is overwhelming. It is important that we care for and about our patients, but I think we can all see the problems that would develop if we suffered alongside them? Back in 2016, Strauss et al. (2016) highlighted the lack of an agreed definition and suggested that without this it would not be possible to 'study compassion, measure compassion or evaluate whether interventions designed to enhance compassion are effective'. In the proceeding years, much scholarly activity has been devoted to addressing this question resulting in a great deal of debate and literature.

There are some points that seem to be common to all definitions, that compassion is 'triggered' by the recognition that a person or group of people are suffering and that the suffering is significant. However, compassion goes beyond recognition (which can result in empathy – the ability to experience and understand a person's experience and feelings) to being motivated to take action to help address a person's suffering. A scoping review by Malenfant et al. (2022) highlights the fact that there continues to be research and discussion about the nature of compassion, so it is clear that the debate about the subject is ongoing. This review did make an important point – that compassion is different from empathy (perhaps the most used alternative word). The difference between the two concepts relates to *action*, empathy compels us to care **about** someone, but compassion compels us to **do** something about their suffering.

West (2021, p. 3) suggested that compassion had four elements:

- Attending (paying attention, being present and noting suffering)
- Understanding (working out what is the cause of the suffering and that this understanding is one that is shared between you and the sufferer)
- Empathising (having felt some connection with the suffering)
- Helping (taking thoughtful and appropriate action to help relieve the suffering).

This can be summed up succinctly in the definition that we can then adopt within this chapter, that compassion is 'a sensitivity to suffering in self and others with a commitment to try to alleviate and prevent it' (Gilbert, 2017).

Activity 8.1   Research and reflection

Type the words 'Courage of Compassion' into your search engine of choice (i.e. Google, DuckDuckGo, or Ecosia) to access the report *The courage of compassion: Supporting nurses and midwives to deliver high-quality care*, written by West, Bailey and Williams in 2020. Scroll to the section that explains what the authors call the 'ABC of nurses' and midwives' core work needs'.

Look at the three sections and the eight associated recommendations made within the report to enable these core work needs to be achieved.

Think about your place of work, consider whether you have access to or have experienced examples of any of these recommendations. Do you think they are realistic? Achievable? Do you think, if implemented, that they would improve your work experience and your ability to provide more compassionate care? If you do not think these recommendations are evident within your workplace, what do you think you could do to encourage implementation?

As this is a reflective activity no model answer is provided; however, some useful resources and ideas are provided at the end of the chapter.

Why does compassion matter?

A true story to illustrate the impact of compassion –

Jane was a teacher and a professional singer, she dealt with the lung cancer that was diagnosed in her late 50s with equanimity and bravery – she would not be defined by it nor let it dominate her life. In hospital following a pneumonectomy that was carried out with the, albeit slim, hope of cure, Jane would recount her experience and tales of the interactions she had with various staff members. The night-time was the thing she dreaded the most. In a side room there was no distraction from either discomfort nor the worries and distress that no matter how well hidden, she inevitably experienced. One nurse responded to her call bell and asked what she needed – Jane explained she was in pain and so the nurse went away and came back promptly with some analgesia. It did not work; Jane remained in pain and rung the bell a number of times throughout the night seeking help. Finally, she even got the feeling that she had been a 'nuisance', she described receiving rather curt and perfunctory treatment.

The following night the situation was the same – she was in pain and so rang her bell. The nurse who responded on this occasion came into the room, stood by the

(Continued)

bed and asked Jane to describe the pain. The nurse asked her if any simple measures such as a position change, rearranging her pillows or making her warmer would be of benefit and did assist her with her pillows. The nurse then told Jane that she had considered what she had been told and what she had observed and that she thought some analgesia would be helpful and that she had identified the appropriate one, the one that she felt would be most effective. Bringing back exactly the same medication as the nurse gave the previous night she stayed while Jane took it, explained that it would not work immediately but that she would check back in about half an hour to see how effective it had been. Leaving Jane with a hot drink – she knew her preference was for black tea – she gave her hand a squeeze, told her she was doing really well in what had been a really difficult time and went back to the other patients. When asked if it had worked, Jane said it must have done because she fell asleep and slept mostly undisturbed until the morning.

It would be easy to reference the evidence base for treating pain as a multi-faceted phenomenon in which analgesia plays only one part in the solution. One could argue that Jane was simply more exhausted the night after the disturbed night previously and that sleep simply overtook her. Or one could acknowledge that she felt seen, she felt safe, and she trusted the nurse to do what she believed to be the right thing for her. It was this, as much if not more, than the analgesia that enabled her to sleep. The benefit of those exquisite, compassionate, sensitive few minutes with Jane was not to her alone – no more call bells summoned anyone that night.

The anthropologist Margaret Mead (1901–1978) suggested that the first evidence of human civilisation was a 15,000-year-old femur bone found in an archaeological dig. The bone showed evidence of having been fractured but also that the fracture had healed, and the person had lived on after the traumatic event that caused the broken bone. In earlier times a wounded person would have been left and would not have survived, but this bone demonstrated that another or others had stayed with the fallen and cared for them until they recovered. The healed femur was a symbol of the transition from a hunter-gatherer lifestyle to a more social, cooperative one – a society where compassion for others was literally lifesaving. While the idea of a healed fracture being the first evidence of human civilisation may be an over-simplification, it highlights the emergence and importance of human empathy and compassion.

Jane's story illustrates how compassion, whilst not lifesaving, did have a significant benefit to the patient and also to the nurses looking after them. A recent increase in research studies looking at the impact of compassionate nursing care on patient outcomes make it increasingly evident that compassionate care provision has a very positive effect on clinical outcomes – compassion is not simply a 'nice' thing to do, compassion is a skill that has significant impact on patient care. A review by Ahmed et al. (2024) found that 'both compassion and transformational leadership can create a positive culture where healthcare professionals prioritise patient safety and quality. Leaders who exhibit compassion are more likely to inspire their teams to deliver patient-centred care and focus on error prevention'. Compassion has been found to reduce the symptoms of depression, anxiety, and psychological distress (Kirby, Tellegen and Steindl, 2017) and increase concordance with treatment (Trzeciak and Mazzarelli, 2019). Robinson et al. (2024) found evidence that compassion improves patient quality of life, hospital experience and overall recovery. So, compassion, far from being a 'soft skill' is a superpower – costing little but impacting hugely, not an option but an imperative.

And compassion benefits not only patients but staff too. Increasingly, burn-out and compassion-fatigue are being linked to the inability of staff to provide care with compassion, to practise in a person-centred way and to form meaningful and satisfying relationships with patients. When the passion most healthcare professionals have for their work is reduced simply to a number of tasks to be achieved, the satisfaction with that work is jeopardised. A study by Chiumento and colleagues (2024) comparing the necessarily functional delivery of care during the COVID-19 pandemic with a more compassionate, person-centred approach demonstrated clear benefit to patients and to the staff who care for them. And, clearly, working in an environment where staff do not get treated with compassion will inevitably impact on their well-being and their willingness to stay within the uncompassionate organisation. As West, Baily and Williams (2020) highlighted, if nurses are enabled to thrive and flourish, they will be better able to provide compassionate, high-quality care.

Assessing and planning based on compassionate principles

The NHS Constitution (2023) establishes the values and principles that underpin care delivery within the NHS in England (the devolved regions of the UK have similar documents). The first statement is that the 'NHS belongs to the people' and that it 'binds together the communities and people it serves'.

Activity 8.2   Reflection

Imagine yourself in the place of the patient, that you have been unwell, are anxious and unsure of what is happening. You meet with an RNA who has been asked to admit you to the hospital. How would you like the RNA to approach you, address you, interact with you? What would be important to you, what would put you at ease and increase your feelings of confidence?

As this is a reflective exercise no model answer is provided.

Empowering patients is a key nursing function and helps to reduce confusion and anxiety; it is therefore important that information is provided at a level and amount that the individual determines. Back in 2010 the then government produced a White Paper (a policy document that outlines proposals for future legislation or action) entitled 'Equity and excellence: Liberating the NHS' which proposed that patients should always be in charge of making decisions about their care. The slogan, *'no decision about me without me'* was included and quoted widely to and by those in charge of the NHS and the direction it was to take. The need to make such a statement seems odd, of course patients should be in charge of their own care...15 years later can we look around us and feel that this really is the case? The nursing workforce cares for the most vulnerable in society – the ill, frightened, confused and suffering. Engaging with the complexity and confusion of healthcare services is challenging enough for those who are well, this is obviously multiplied when the person is struggling with ill health. Person-centredness will not happen by chance, it takes commitment, effort and a culture that supports and promotes this approach – a culture based on compassion.

Activity 8.3   Critical thinking

An RNA is working in a busy Emergency Department, over the course of their shift they meet many different patients. Emily is an 82-year-old lady who is brought in by ambulance following a fall in the care home where she lives, she has dementia. Joshua is three and has bronchiolitis, he comes in with his parents and is well known to the paediatric team. Emma is 46 and has Down's Syndrome, she is known to have pulmonary hypertension and has come to ED with her care worker as she has had a cold recently and has been getting increasingly short of breath.

In order to ensure that each of these people receive compassionate, person-centred assessment and subsequent treatment, what document(s) would you look for that may accompany them? Why and by whom have these documents been developed?

A model answer is provided at the end of the chapter.

Compassion requires us to be present with people, to hear what they say, to be honest – gently so where necessary – and to ensure that their plan of care reflects their individual needs. This can seem like a difficult task when time and resources are in short supply, and it is easy to understand why healthcare can become 'task-oriented' rather than 'people-oriented'. However, here's the thing – if we get it right first time and align 'our' plans with the individual person's plans and needs then this can often save time in the longer term. Lord Darzi (Department of Health, 2024) makes it clear that improvements are needed within the NHS and that, 'the best change empowers patients to take as much control of their care as possible'.

Understand the theory

The Mental Capacity Act (2005) is an important guide which sets out the requirement to advocate for and empower people to make their own decisions. It contains five key main principles:

1. Presumption of Capacity – you must presume people have the capacity to make their own decisions unless you are able to demonstrate that they cannot. A lack of capacity should not automatically be assumed simply based on a person's age, appearance, condition or behaviour.
2. Support to make decisions – you must make every effort to help people make their own decisions – the responsibility lies with the health professionals and includes providing information, access to communication aids, assessing understanding.
3. Ability to make unwise decisions – just because a person does not follow advice or do what you think best does not mean that they lack capacity.
4. Best interests – if someone cannot make their own decisions then the decisions made on their behalf must be in their best interests. This means considering their wishes, past and present, as well as their well-being and any other relevant factors.

(Continued)

(Continued)

5. Least restrictive option – if a person lacks capacity and needs a decision made in their best interests this should be the least restrictive option possible emphasising the person's rights and freedoms.

You need to be aware of these five principles, an Act of Parliament creates a new law or changes an existing one – it is therefore a legal requirement to follow the principles of the Mental Capacity Act. The principles of this Act demand of us that we place the patient at the centre of their care, it is inherently compassionate and person-centred and MUST underpin how you assess a patient's needs and plan and evaluate their care.

How compassionate cultures ensure compassionate care

The idea that being polite can have a profound impact on patient care could sound rather farfetched if taken simply at face value. However, the movement 'Civility Saves Lives' exists to raise awareness of the significance that behaviour has on well-being, performance and, ultimately, patient safety. Previously, in this book and much more extensively in 'Team Working and Professional Practice' (Bibi, Comley and Forman, 2022) the importance of effective teamworking to deliver safe and effective care has been explored and described. Put simply, poor teams provide poor care, and poor care can endanger patients' lives, so how a team performs is vitally important. A survey carried out by West and Dawson for the King's Fund as far back as 2012 discovered that when staff believed they were part of a good team they experienced the following benefits:

- Reduced mortality rates
- Reduced patient complaints
- Improved staff satisfaction
- Improved staff performance
- Better reported staff health

So, civility, like compassion, has a direct impact on not just the outcome for the patients but also for the well-being of the staff looking after them.

Activity 8.4   Reflective practice

Access the Civility Saves Lives website on www.civilitysaveslives.com and scroll to the bottom of the Home page where you will find a 15-minute TEDx video entitled 'When rudeness in teams turns deadly' by Chris Turner.

Think about the last few weeks when you have been working in your job as a SNA or as an RNA, what behaviours have you witnessed by colleagues (or even yourself. . .) that you believe lacked civility (or kindness or compassion)? They could be subtle (such as eye rolling or tutting) or more significant (raised voices, unkind comments) – there are many ways that these behaviours are demonstrated, and they could have been directed at you or at or about others. How were you left feeling? How did your opinion about your colleague alter, if it did? What impact did experiencing this have on the rest of your day and your feelings about your next shift? Did watching the TEDx video remind you of experiences you have had? Were you surprised at how significant even witnessing incivility can be?

There are so many things to think about after watching the video, some will be addressed by the specific questions above, but, take your time to reflect and consider and think how you might want to change your own thinking or, even, behaviour.

As this is a reflective exercise no model answer is provided but some additional resources can be found at the end of the chapter.

A lot of the theory relating to civility and the impact this can have on individuals and teams has been published by Christine Porath, an Associate Professor of Management at a University in America. Her work is relevant to all areas where people work together in teams (almost everywhere) and very much so when the output of that team is human health and life.

So, what is incivility?

It is obvious really as it boils down to any behaviour that causes a negative emotion in another, importantly it is how the *recipient* experiences it that will define it as uncivil. So, someone may not believe or intend their behaviour to negatively impact another but, if it does, then the behaviour may well need addressing. Examples, by no way exhaustive, of rude behaviour could include: shouting at someone, using bad language, sending emails or using a computer during meetings, criticising someone, talking over others or ignoring their input, being curt or dismissive on the phone (not my problem?), tutting, laughing at someone….the list goes on.

Look at the infographic below (Figure 8.1), the figures are stark and clearly illustrate how damaging rudeness can be.

This is startling enough, but this is not the only research that demonstrates the impact of rudeness. Riskin et al. (2015) showed that medical staff exposed to a mildly rude comment in a neonatal intensive care simulation had a 20 per cent drop in their clinical performance and a 50 per cent reduction in behaviours such as information sharing and seeking help.

And, as students who are training and educating themselves to be the healthcare professionals of the future? Cheetham and Turner (2020) found that incivility had a negative impact on learning and recall. So, it is important that educators also create supportive, kind and civil environments in which students are enabled to learn to their highest potential.

And why is this so important when considering the assessment, planning and evaluation of a person's care? Well, failure to engage with the patient you are assessing, failure to form a meaningful relationship and to demonstrate that you care and are interested in them is likely to have a negative impact on the depth, accuracy and relevance of the assessment. And, if this initial part of the patient journey is not well managed, the potential is for all subsequent steps to be compromised. Patients who do not feel listened to or cared about are unlikely to feel so comfortable sharing information, confiding in you, to do as you suggest (being concordant) or readily getting in touch in the future if they are worried. Any of these elements alone can impact the outcome of a patient's care, all together and the negative connotations are obvious. So, being compassionate, civil and listening to people isn't just a decent and humane way to interact with patients, it is a clinically effective skill to ensure best possible outcomes.

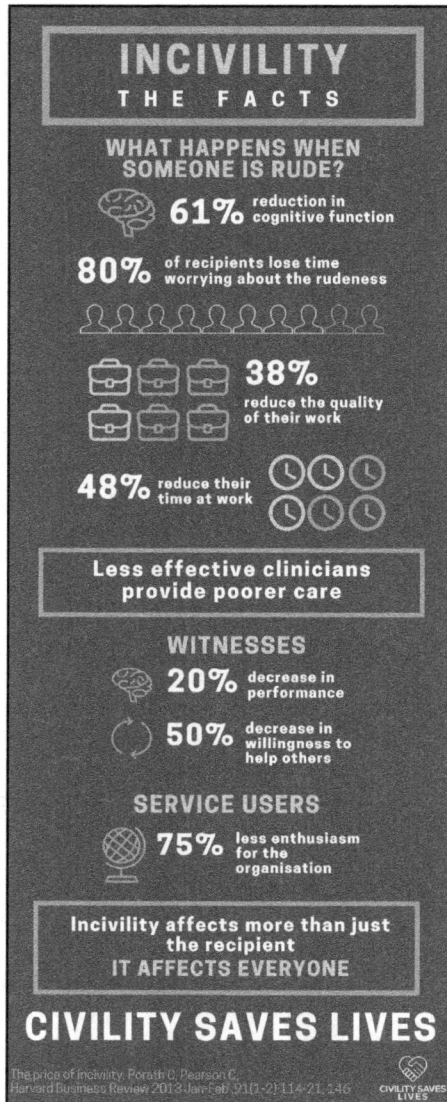

Figure 8.1 Civility saves lives

Source: www.civilitysaveslives.com/infographics

When compassion is especially important – when there may be no second chance to get it right

All people deserve to be treated with compassion, to have a person-centred and holistic assessment and a plan of care tailored to their needs as far as is possible. However, there is an especially compelling need to get this right when caring for those who are approaching the end of their lives – get things wrong at this point and there may be little, if any, opportunity to correct the error.

Advance decision

In some circumstances, patients will anticipate their future care needs and might create a document known as an 'Advance decision to refuse treatment' – also sometimes known as a 'living will'. This document enables a person to make it clear which medical treatments they do or do not want to be given by healthcare staff. As long as the decision is clear, the circumstances when it needs to be adhered to are specific and the decision was made by a person with capacity as per the Mental Capacity Act (2005) then it is legally binding.

Whilst this document is designed to provide information to a healthcare team about a person's wishes in situations where they are no longer able to express themselves it can also serve other functions. An Advance Decision may also prevent confusion and disagreement between healthcare teams or between healthcare staff and a patient's next-of-kin – knowing the patient's clear and documented wishes prevents potentially stressful situations intruding on what should be a time of peace and dignity. Patients report finding it stressful having to keep repeating information, especially very emotive or distressing information, to the numerous healthcare professionals they encounter. An Advanced Directive may prevent the need to continually repeat themselves, although it is important to check that the details of the Advanced Directive still reflect the person's wishes.

Understand the theory

The NHS states that:

An advance decision (sometimes known as an advance decision to refuse treatment, an ADRT, or a living will) is a decision you can make now to refuse a specific type of treatment at some time in the future.

It lets your family, carers and health professionals know your wishes about refusing treatment if you're unable to make or communicate those decisions yourself.

The treatments you're deciding to refuse must all be named in the advance decision.

You may want to refuse a treatment in some situations, but not others. If this is the case, you need to be clear about all the circumstances in which you want to refuse this treatment.

You can refuse a treatment that could potentially keep you alive, known as life-sustaining treatment.

This is treatment that replaces or supports ailing bodily functions, such as:

- Ventilation – this may be used if you cannot breathe by yourself
- Cardiopulmonary resuscitation (CPR) – this may be used if your heart stops
- Antibiotics – this can help your body fight infection

You make the advance decision, as long as you have the mental capacity to make such decisions.

If you decide to refuse life-sustaining treatment in the future, your advance decision needs to be:

- Written down
- Signed by you
- signed by a witness

If you wish to refuse life-sustaining treatments in circumstances where you might die as a result, you need to state this clearly in your advance decision. Life-sustaining treatment is sometimes called life-saving treatment.

An advance decision is legally binding as long as it:

(Continued)

(Continued)
- Complies with the Mental Capacity Act
- Is valid
- Applies to the situation

If your advance decision is binding, it takes precedence over decisions made in your best interest by other people.

An advance decision may only be considered valid if:

- You're aged 18 years old or over and had the capacity to make, understand, and communicate your decision when you made it;
- You specify clearly which treatments you wish to refuse;
- You explain the circumstances in which you wish to refuse them;
- It's signed by you (and by a witness if you want to refuse life-sustaining treatment);
- You have made the advance decision of your own accord, without any harassment by anyone else;
- You have not said or done anything that would contradict the advance decision since you made it (for example, saying that you've changed your mind).

As well as an Advance Decision, a person can also have an Advance Statement, this document enables more general points to be recorded. An Advance Statement might describe religious or other beliefs, wishes that reflect important aspects of a person's life such as family input, dietary preferences, care of pets or even what clothes or television programmes someone prefers. The most important thing is to check – check what the person wants, check how they can let you know, check if they have any advance directives or statements.

Case study 8.1 Peter

Chris is an SNA on placement with a community nursing team and is accompanying Sonia, the Team Leader on a visit to the home of Peter, a 52-year-old man who has Motor Neurone Disease (MND). The team have been looking after Peter for over a year and know him well, he lives at home with the help and care of his long-term partner Darren. The nurses call regularly and help with supplementary feeding via a percutaneous endoscopic gastrostomy (PEG) tube, support for his breathing via non-invasive ventilation (NIV) and pressure area care as Peter is becoming increasingly immobile and is now totally reliant on a hoist and a wheelchair to get about. Following a recent chest infection which was treated with antibiotics, Peter's overall condition has noticeably declined. He is due to be admitted to the local hospital for assessment and the consideration of increased levels of support including moving to all food and fluids via PEG, the possibility of invasive ventilation via tracheostomy and a discussion with the specialist psychologist.

Peter has a good relationship with Sonia and has specifically requested that she come and visit him as he needs some help. On arrival Sonia checks with Peter and Darren that they are happy for Chris to be there, Darren appears distressed, but both agree to Chris being present. Everyone sits in the lounge; Peter is in his wheelchair with the NIV face mask in place and says that although the mask was usually only used at night, he is now finding it increasingly difficult to manage without it. As he has the mask on, he cannot easily eat and drink and, when he does try the small amount of food he used to enjoy he now frequently chokes which he finds very frightening. His speech is slow and difficult to understand and as he is talking Darren sits with tears streaming down his face. Peter tells Sonia that he does not want to go into hospital, that he has had enough and cannot see any future that he would find tolerable. He wants to compile an Advance Decision document but wants some advice as Darren finds the idea too distressing even though he says he will go along with whatever Peter wants.

Activity 8.5   Critical thinking

In response to the case study above:

- What could Sonia do in this circumstance?
- Is it acceptable for her to help Peter to create an Advance Decision?
- What would she need to assess?
- What resources could she use to help support Peter and Darren?
- What would she need to consider about her and Chris?

A model answer with some suggested responses is included at the end of the chapter.

Lasting power of attorney

Wherever possible an individual must be supported to make decisions for themselves; however, some people will plan for the possibility that they may one day be unable to make their wishes known. As with the Advance Decision, appointing someone as a Lasting Power of Attorney (LPA) aims to ensure that your wishes can be known even if you are not able to express them yourself. An LPA identifies a person (a relative, friend, partner, or a professional such as a solicitor) that you appoint to make decisions on your behalf, known as an attorney. The LPA is a legal document that has to be completed when you have capacity, and which requires witnesses and a 'certificate provider' who confirms that you do have capacity and are not under duress. The LPA then has to be registered with the Office of the Public Guardian, the process can take a number of weeks to complete.

There are two types of LPA – for health and welfare and for property and financial affairs. If an attorney is appointed LPA for health and welfare and the person who has appointed them no longer has capacity or is too ill to make their wishes known, then the attorney has the power to make significant decisions such as the provision of life-sustaining treatment or moving into residential care. It is an important role and healthcare staff must ask to see the evidence that the attorney does hold an LPA, once this is established then the LPA speaks for and AS the patient. For nurses, establishing if someone does have an LPA is important as this person can help provide the necessary information to ensure accurate assessment and person-centred planning.

Activity 8.6   Research

Sonia and Chris (see Case study 8.1) are made aware that Darren was appointed as a Lasting Power of Attorney for health and well-being by Peter when he was first diagnosed with MND.

Access the UK government website www.gov.uk/power-of-attorney and read the information about how an attorney is appointed and what needs to happen when someone holds an LPA. Once you have read this information you can reconsider your answer to Activity 8.5 and add any further details that you feel might be helpful.

A model answer is included at the end of the chapter.

It goes without saying that people and their loved ones who are being cared for in the final stages of their lives need sensitive, skilled and compassionate care. In 2008, the NHS developed the first strategy for end-of-life care in England; subsequently, the NHS joined with a large body of other statutory and voluntary organisations to create the National Palliative and End of Life Care Partnership. In 2021, this organisation set out a national framework and stated that 'how we care for the dying is an indicator of how we care for all sick and vulnerable people'. In 2015, The National Institute for Health and Care Excellence (NICE) published guidelines to ensure that the final days of a person's life are supported and managed to the best possible standards. All of these key documents emphasise the importance of personalised assessment and planning to ensure people receive the care that they need. Care provided with compassion not only helps to ensure the most peaceful and symptom-free death possible for the patient, it can also help the onward journey of those bereaved by the loss of their loved one.

Why does compassion matter #2

The true story continues and serves to illustrate how simple acts can have a profound impact:

Unfortunately, despite the extensive surgery that Jane underwent to try and cure the lung cancer she had been diagnosed with, the disease returned. Jane underwent various regimes of chemotherapy and radiotherapy and endured all stoically and with great positivity, she made it clear that she would not be defined by the illness. Jane continued to work as a teacher, she sang in a concert to raise money for the local chemotherapy unit and set about living her life. Eventually, even her indefatigable nature was overwhelmed by the cancer and she returned home from hospital to a package of care and the support of her family and friends for her final weeks.

During one visit by the domiciliary carers, Jane was sleeping peacefully and her partner and friends said that they had recently changed her position, so nothing

(Continued)

was needed at that time. One of the carers, who had been a number of times previously, noted the musical instruments that were all around the house, including a piano in the lounge where Jane was sleeping in a hospital bed. The carer asked if she could use the time instead to play for Jane. In the half an hour that followed Jane slept on gently, her partner, several family members and friends sat together – all present and 'held' by the soft and tranquil music. It was a shared moment of stillness, a gift in a time of sadness and loss and it is a memory that still provides comfort and grace over a decade later to those who were present.

Conclusion

Compassion is an approach to patient care, to assessment, planning and evaluation, that needs consideration and intent. Many healthcare professionals have the capacity and innate ability to provide compassionate care, all have the potential to do so (the definition of a person without compassion is a psychopath!) However, even the most compassionate person will struggle to provide compassionate care if they work in an environment and culture where compassion is not valued, not modelled and not mandated. As with all 'movements' it takes individuals to identify their priorities and values, they then influence followers who join together and influence others until – the movement is unstoppable!

So, be the person who believes that assessment is more than a series of drop-down boxes, sit beside the patient and listen to what they say, plan care that matters to the recipient and ensure that care is regularly evaluated and updated. 'Wear' your compassion proudly and use the language of evidence to promote compassion – not simply as a human thing to do but as a clinically relevant and important element of effective patient care. This chapter can only introduce you to concepts and ideas, so if you think the points raised are important then read, explore and discover more for yourself. The power of compassion, of civility, of empathy to have a clinical impact on patient outcomes is attracting more and more attention, make sure that you keep up with this important element of practice.

Chapter summary

This chapter has focused on the importance of compassion as an underpinning element of the provision of effective assessment, planning and evaluation of care. The challenge of definition was described along with a chosen definition to support the points within this chapter. Compassionate cultures and the impact on staff and patient were explored as well as the impact of individuals to the development of a compassionate workplace. The importance of compassion for those who are reaching the end of their lives and how this also influences the care that all patients receive was highlighted. A true story of one, ordinary individual was used to illustrate the impact of compassion, to provide a way of citing the theory described within the chapter firmly within the realities of patient care.

Activities: Brief outline answers and useful resources

Activity 8.1 Research and reflection (page 126)

This is the website address for the report *The courage of compassion: Supporting nurses and midwives to deliver high-quality care 2020:* www.kingsfund.org.uk/insight-and-analysis/reports/courage-compassion-supporting-nurses-midwives#personal-impact-and-influence-programme.

This is a really interesting article about how nurses can take action to improve the culture in nursing – Bosanquet, J. (2021) Providing not prescribing: fostering a culture of wellbeing in nursing. *Journal of Research in Nursing,* 26(5): 367–375.

Activity 8.3 Critical thinking (page 129)

There are a number of different personalised documents that can accompany anyone who may have difficulties explaining their individual preferences and needs. The Alzheimer's Society has developed a 'Forget Me Not' document which includes details about a person's likes and dislikes, routines, family circumstances and preferences for how they are addressed and how to communicate effectively with them. Many Trusts will have a version of this form, it is often called 'This is Me' or perhaps 'My Care Passport' or 'Hospital Passport' and provides a similar opportunity to record preferences. Versions of the document exist that are tailored to the needs of children and their families (e.g., www.togetherforshortlives.org.uk/resource/editable-hospital-passport-template/) and for those who have a learning disability (see www.mefirst.org.uk/resource/hospital-passport/). If a person is to receive compassionate care, then it MUST be based on their individual needs and preferences – it is the health professionals' obligation to establish what these are by any and all means possible.

Activity 8.4 Reflective practice (page 130)

As well as the Civility Saves Lives website, this blog from The Queen's Nursing Institute in Scotland is interesting www.qnis.org.uk/blog/civility-saves-lives-why-how-we-treat-each-other-really-matters/

The NHS has developed a toolkit to help staff develop cultures where civility and respect underpin teams and service provision – available at:www.socialpartnershipforum.org/system/files/2021-10/NHSi-Civility-and-Respect-Toolkit-v9.pdf.

Activity 8.5 Case study

Sonia will undoubtedly be challenged to be faced with such a situation, so she would need to take her time to find out what has brought Peter to this decision. Is this a deeply held and final decision or a reaction to his recent deterioration? Sonia would need to establish that he has the capacity to make such a decision. Grief and loss are not just a reaction to death, patients also feel these emotions when faced with loss of health, independence, future plans – such grief can impact a person's capacity. So, Sonia would need the help of other healthcare professionals who may know Peter – his GP, the Consultant Neurologist, the MND Nurse Specialist, an appropriate Psychologist, staff or patients from the local MND charity, perhaps a religious representative if Peter has a faith. It is certainly within Sonia's remit to assist Peter with creating an Advanced

Directive but before doing so Sonia would need to seek support and advice too. Finally, such an emotive and distressing meeting would have impact; both on Sonia and on Chris, so time to reflect, debrief and get/give support would be important.

Activity 8.6 Research (page 136)

The answer above does not change however, as an attorney for health and well-being, Darren would need to be aware of any decisions and choices that Peter makes. Whilst he has the capacity to make decisions, Peter remains in charge of the direction that his care takes. However, were his condition to deteriorate to the extent that he was no longer able to make his wishes known, Darren would speak on his behalf. It is therefore important that Darren understands and is happy to support Peter's wishes, if he does not agree or feels conflicted in any way then he would need to make his concerns known and Peter could appoint a different attorney.

References

Ahmed, Z., Ellahham, S., Soomro, M., Shams, S. and Latif, K. (2024). Exploring the impact of compassion and leadership on patient safety and quality in healthcare systems: A narrative review. *BMJ Open Quality*, 13:e002651. https://doi.org/10.1136/ bmjoq-2023-002651

Airedale NHS Trust v Bland. (1993). 1 All ER 821. https://www.globalhealthrights.org/wp-content/uploads/2013/01/HL-1993-Airedale-NHS-Trust-v.-Bland.pdf (Accessed 15 October 2025).

Aldridge, J. (2004). Learning disability nursing: A model for practice. In: Turnbull J. (ed) *Learning Disability Nursing*. Oxford: Blackwell Science.

Anandarajah, G. and Hight, E. (2001). Spirituality and medical practice: Using the HOPE questions as a practical tool for spiritual assessment. *American Family Physician*, 63(1):81–89.

Atkinson, D., Boulter, P., Hebron, C., Moulster, G. (2013). The Health Equalities Framework (HEF). An outcomes framework based on the determinants of health inequalities: A Guide for Practitioners.

Bapen. (2003). *Malnutrition universal screening tool*. Available online: www.bapen.org.uk/pdfs/must/must_full.pdf

Barker, P. J. and Buchanan-Barker, P. (2005). *The tidal model: A guide for mental health professionals*. Hove England: Brunner-Routledge.

Barnardo's. (2024). Changing childhoods. *Changing lives*. https://cms.barnardos.org.uk/sites/default/files/2024-03/Changing%20Childhoods%20Changing%20Lives%20Report_Digital.pdf

BBC News. (2020). *Ella Adoo-Kissi-Debrah: Air pollution a factor in girl's death, inquest finds*. Available online: www.bbc.co.uk/news/uk-england-london-55330945

Beauchamp, T. L. and Childress, J. F. (1979). *Principles of biomedical ethics*. New York: Oxford University Press.

Beauchamp, T. L. and Childress, J. F. (2019). *Principles of biomedical ethics 8th edition*. New York: Oxford University Press.

Benner, P. (1982). From novice to expert. *The American Journal of Nursing*, 82(3):402–407.

Benner, P. (1984). *From novice to expert: Excellence and power in clinical nursing practice*. Menlo Park: Addison-Wesley.

Bieri, D., Reeve, R. A, Champion, G. D., Addicoat, L. and Ziegler, J. B. (1990). The faces pain scale for the self-assessment of the severity of pain experienced by children: Development, initial validation and preliminary investigation for ration scale properties. *Pain*, 41:139–150.

Blanks, R. G., Wallis, M. G., and Moss, S. M. (1998). A comparison of cancer detection rates achieved by breast cancer screening programmes by number of readers, for one and two view mammography: Results from the UK National Health Service breast screening programme. *Journal of Medical Screening*, 5(4):195–201.

British Medical Association. (2004). *Assessment of mental capacity: Guidance for doctors and lawyers*. BMJ Books.

Cambridge University Press. (n.d.) Available at: https://dictionary.cambridge.org/dictionary/english/teamwork (Accessed 24 October 2024).

References

Casey, A. (1988). A partnership with child and family. *Senior Nurse*, 8(4):8–9.

Cheetham, L. J. E. and Turner, C. (2020) Incivility and the clinical learner. *Future Healthcare Journal*, 7(2):109–111.

Chiumento, A., Fovargue, S., Redhead, C., Draper, H. and Frith, L. (2024) Delivering compassionate NHS healthcare: A qualitative study exploring the ethical implications of resetting NHS maternity and paediatric services following the acute phase of the COVID-19 pandemic. *Social Science & Medicine*, 344:116503. https://doi.org/10.1016/j.socscimed.2023.116503

Collins English Dictionary. (n.d.). *Tool.* Available online: www.collinsdictionary.com/dictionary/english/tool (Accessed 08 June 2025).

Collins Dictionary (n.d.). Available at: www.collinsdictionary.com/english-language-learning/intuition#google_vignette (Accessed 08 June 2025).

Coulter, A. and Collins, A. (2011). *Making shared decision-making a reality. No decision about me, without me.* King's Fund.

Cox, J. L., Holdenm, J. M. and Sagovsky, R. (1987). Detection of postnatal depression. Development of the 10-item Edinburgh postnatal depression scale. *The British Journal of Psychiatry*, 150:782–786. PMID:3651732

Dahlgren, G. and Whitehead, M. (2021).The Dahlgren-Whitehead model of health determinants: 30 years on and still chasing rainbows. *Public Health*, 199:20–24.

Department of Health. (2011). No health without mental health: A cross-government mental health outcomes strategy for people of all ages. *No Health Without Mental Health: A cross-government outcomes strategy - GOV.UK.*

Department of Health. (2023). *The NHS constitution for England.* Online. Available at: www.gov.uk/government/publications/the-nhs-constitution-for-england/the-nhs-constitution-for-england

Department of Health. (2024). *Independent investigation of the NHS in England Lord Darzi's report on the state of the National Health Service in England.* Online. Available at: www.gov.uk/government/publications/independent-investigation-of-the-nhs-in-england

Department of Health and Social Care. (2024). *Hospital discharge and community support guidance.* Available online: www.gov.uk/government/publications/hospital-discharge-and-community-support-guidance/hospital-discharge-and-community-support-guidance#about-this-guidance

Department of Health and Social Care. (2024). *Summary letter from Lord Darzi to the secretary of state for health and social care.* www.gov.uk/government/publications/independent-investigation-of-the-nhs-in-england/summary-letter-from-lord-darzi-to-the-secretary-of-state-for-health-and-social-care (Accessed 17 November 2024).

Dreyfus, S. E. (1981). Four models v human situational understanding: Inherent limitations on the modelling of business expertise USAF Office of Scientific Research, ref F49620-79-C-0063.

Ellis, P., Standing, M. and Roberts, S. (2020). *Patient assessment & care planning in nursing.* London: Sage Publishing.

Emerson, E. and Baines, S. (2011). Health inequalities and people with learning disabilities in the UK: 2011. *Learning Disabilities Public Health Observatory.*

Equality Act. (2010). Legislation.gov.uk. Available from: www.gov.uk/guidance/equality-act-2010-guidance (Accessed 31 March 2025).

Ferraz, M. B., Quaresma, M. R., Aquino, L. R., Atra, E., Tugwell, P. and Goldsmith, C. H. (August 1990). Reliability of pain scales in the assessment of literate and illiterate patients with rheumatoid arthritis. *The Journal of Rheumatology*, 17(8):1022–1024.

Garra, G., Singer, A. J., Taira, B. R., Chohan, J., Cardoz, H., Chisena, E. and Thode, H. C. (2010). Validation of the wong-baker FACES pain scale in pediatric emergency department patients. *Academic Emergency Medicine*, 17(1):50–54.

Gibbs, G. (1988). *Learning by doing: A guide to teaching and learning methods*. Oxford: Further Education Unit, Oxford Polytechnic.

Gilbert, P. (Ed.) (2017). *Compassion: Definitions and controversies in compassion: Concepts, research and applications*. Oxford: Routledge.

Gilhooly, D., Green, S. A., McCann, C., Black, N. and Moonesinghe, S. R. (2019). Barriers and facilitators to the successful development, implementation and evaluation of care bundles in acute care in hospital: A scoping review. *Implementation Science*, 14:47. https://doi.org/ 10.1186/s13012-019-0894-2

Glasper, A. (2020). Strategies to ensure that all patients have a personalised nursing care plan. *British Journal of Nursing*, 29(1):62–63.

Halloran, E. J. (1996). Virginia Henderson and her timeless writings. *Journal of Advanced Nursing*, 23:17–27.

Hammond, K. R. (1981). *Principles of organization in intuitive and analytical cognition*. University of Colorado.

Hams, P. S. (2000). A gut feeling? Intuition and critical care nursing. *Journal of Intensive and Critical Care Nursing*, 16:310–318.

Harris, M. (2021) *Understanding person-centred care for nursing associates*. London: Learning Matters: Sage Publishing Co.

Heath and Care Act. (2022). c. 31 available at: www.legislation.gov.uk/ukpga/2022/31/contents

Health Education England. (2021). *Working differently together: Progressing a one workforce approach*. Multidisciplinary team toolkit. www.hee.nhs.uk/sites/default/files/documents/ HEE_MDT_Toolkit_V1.1.pdf

The Health Foundation. (2016). *Person-centred care made simple: What everyone should know about person-centred care*. London: The Health Foundation.

The Health Foundation. (2018). *Living alone matters: Linking data to explore the connection between older people living alone and A&E attendance*. Available online: www.health.-org.uk/features-and-opinion/blogs/living-alone-matters#:~:text=Living%20alone%20can%20increase%20a,smoking%2015%20cigarettes%20a%20day

The Health Foundation. (2023a). *Health in 20240: Projected patterns of illness in England*. www.health.org.uk/reports-and-analysis/reports/health-in-2040-projected-patterns-of-illness-in-england

The Health Foundation. (2023b). *Briefing: Realising the potential of community-based multidisciplinary teams. Insight from Evidence*. London: The Health Foundation.

Huesmann, L., Sudacka, M., Durning, S. J., Georg, C., Huwendiek, S., Kononowicz, A. A. and Hege, I. (2023). Clinical reasoning: What do nurses, physicians, and students reason about. *Journal of Interprofessional Care*, 37(6): 990–998. https://doi.org/10.1080/ 13561820.2023.2208605

Henderson, V. (1969). *Basic principles of nursing care*. Geneva: International Council of Nurses.

Holland, K. (2008). *Applying the Roper-Logan-Tierney model in practice*. Edinburgh: Churchill Livingstone.

Iohom, G. (2006). Chapter 11 - Clinical assessment of postoperative pain. In: Shorten, G., Carr, D. B., Harmon, D., Puig, M. M., Browne, J. (eds) *Postoperative Pain Management*, W.B. Saunders, pp. 102–108. ISBN 9781416024545.

Iragorri, N. and Spackman, E. (2018). Assessing the value of screening tools: Reviewing the challenges and opportunities of cost-effectiveness analysis. *Public Health Reviews*, 39:17. https://doi.org/10.1186/s40985-018-0093-8

Joint Formulary Committee. (2025). *Iodine*. Available online: https://bnf.nice.org.uk/drugs/ iodide-with-iodine/#side-effects (Accessed 08 June 2025).

Kahneman, D. (2011). *Thinking, fast and slow*. Doubleday Canada.

Kirby, J. N., Tellegen, C. L. and Steindl, S. R. (2017). A meta-analysis of compassion-based interventions: Current state of knowledge and future directions. *Behavioural Therapy*, 48: 778–792.

Kroenke, K., Spitzer, R. L., Williams, J. B., Monahan, P. O. and Löwe, B. (6 March 2007). Anxiety disorders in primary care: Prevalence, impairment, comorbidity, and detection. *Annals of Internal Medicine*, 146(5):317–325. https://doi.org/10.7326/0003-4819-146-5-200703060-00004. PMID: 17339617.

Kroenke, K., Spitzer, R. L. and William, J. B. (2001). The PHQ-9: Validity of a brief severity depression measure. *Journal of General Internal Medicine*, 16(9):606–613.

Lancman, B., Jorm, C., Iedema, R., Piper, D. and Manidis, M. (2015). Taking the heat in critical situations: Being aware, assertive and heard. *Communicating Quality and Safety in Health Care*, 2015:268–279.

Lazaridou, A., Elbaridi, N., Edwards, R. R. and Berde, C. B. (2018). Chapter 5 - Pain assessment. In H. T. Benzon, S. N. Raja, S. S. Liu, S. M. Fishman, S. P. Cohen (eds) *Essentials of Pain Medicine* (Fourth Edition), Elsevier, 2018:39–46. e1.

LeDeR. (2023). *Learning disability mortality review: Annual report*. NHS. Bristol, North Somerset, and South Gloucestershire Integrated Care Board.

Levett-Jones, T., Hoffman, K., Dempsey, J., Yeun-Sim Jeong, S., Noble, D., Norton, C. A., Roche, J. and Hickey, N. (2010). The 'five rights' of clinical reasoning: An educational model to enhance nursing students' ability to identify and manage clinically 'at risk' patients. *Nurse Education Today*, 30(6):515–520.

Malenfant, S., Jaggi, P., Hayden, K. A. and Sinclair, S. (2022). Compassion in healthcare: An updated scoping review of the literature. *BMC Palliative Care*, 21:80.

Margolis, C. Z. (1983) Uses of Clinical Algorithms. *JAMA: The Journal of the American Medical Association*, 249(5): 627–632.

Marmot, M., Allen, J., Goldblatt, P., Boyce, T., McNeish, D., Grady, M. and Geddes, I. (2010). *Fair society, healthy lives: The marmot review*. Available online: www.parliament.uk/global-assets/documents/fair-society-healthy-lives-full-report.pdf

Marmot, M., Allen, J., Boyce, T., Goldblatt, P. and Morrison, J. (2020). *Health inequality in England: The marmot review 10 years on*. Available online: www.instituteofhealthequity.org/resources-reports/marmot-review-10-years-on/the-marmot-review-10-years-on-full-report.pdf

McCormack, B. and McCance, T. (2006). Development of a framework for person-centred nursing. *Journal of Advanced Nursing*, 56:472–479. https://doi.org/10.1111/j.1365-2648.2006.04042.x

McKenna, H. P. (1997). *Nursing theories and models*. New York, NY: Routledge.

Melzack, R. (1975). The McGill pain questionnaire: Major properties and scoring methods. *Pain*, 1(3):277–299.

Melzack R. (August 1987). The short-form McGill pain questionnaire. *Pain*, 30(2):191–197. https://doi.org/10.1016/0304-3959(87)91074-8. PMID: 3670870.

Mental Capacity Act. (2005). Legislation.gov.uk. Mental Capacity Act 2005, c. 9. Available at: https://www.legislation.gov.uk/ukpga/2005/9/contents

Merriam-Webster. (n.d.). Compassion. In *Merriam-Webster.com dictionary*. Retrieved 6 May 2025, from https://www.merriam-webster.com/dictionary/compassion

Moulster, G., Ames, S., Lorrizo, J. and Kernohan, J. (2019). A flexible model to support person-centred learning disability nursing. *Nursing Times*, 115(6):56–59.

National Health Service. (2021). *NHS screening*. Available at: www.nhs.uk/conditions/nhs-screening/

National Health Service. (2022). *Paediatric acute abdominal pain and appendicectomy: Best practice pathway guidance*.

National Health Service, The. (2010). *National end of life care programme: Improving end of life care.*

National Health Service. (2024). *Workforce, training and education: Person-centred care.* Available online at: www.hee.nhs.uk/our-work/person-centred-care (last accessed 7 May 2024).

National Institute for Health and Care Excellence. (2024). *Suspected sepsis: Recognition, diagnosis and early management.* Available at: www.nice.org.uk/guidance/NG51

National Institute for Health and Care Excellence. (2024). *Clinical skills summary how should i assess a person's risk of developing a pressure ulcer?* Available online: https://cks.nice.org.uk/topics/pressure-ulcers/diagnosis/risk-assessment/ (Accessed 08 June 2025).

National Institute for Health and Care Excellence. (2015). *Care of dying adults in the last days of life.* NICE guideline: Reference number:NG31.

National Palliative and End of Life Care Partnership. (2021). *Ambitions for Palliative and End of Life Care: A national framework for local action 2021-2026.* [Online] Available at: www.england.nhs.uk/wp-content/uploads/2022/02/ambitions-for-palliative-and-end-of-life-care-2nd-edition.pdf

NHS England. (2019). *Learning Disability Mortality Review (LeDeR) Programme.* Available at https://www.england.nhs.uk/wp-content/uploads/2019/05/action-from-learning.pdf

NHS England and the Department of Health and Social Care. (2022). *Working in partnership with people and communities: Statutory guidance.* https://www.england.nhs.uk/wp-content/uploads/2023/05/B1762-guidance-on-working-in-partnership-with-people-and-communities-2.pdf (Accessed 19 November 2024).

NHS England. (2019). *The NHS long term plan.* Available at: www.longtermplan.nhs.uk/wp-content/uploads/2019/01/nhs-long-term-plan-june-2019.pdf

NHS England. (2020). *The NHS people plan 2020/21.* Available at: www.england.nhs.uk/wp-content/uploads/2020/07/We-Are-The-NHS-Action-For-All-Of-Us-FINAL-March-21.pdf

NHS England. (2024). *Person-centered care.* NHS.

NHS England. (2019). *Comprehensive model for personalised care.* Available at: www.england.nhs.uk/publication/comprehensive-model-of-personalised-care/

Nibbelink, C. W. and Brewer, B. B. (2018). Decision-making in nursing practice: An integrative literature review. *Journal of Clinical Nursing,* 27(5–6):917–928. https://doi.org/10.1111/jocn.14151

NICE. (2016). *Mental health problems in people with learning disabilities: Prevention, assessment, and management.* NICE guideline (NG54).

Nursing and Midwifery Council. (2018). *The code: Professional standards of practice and behaviour for nurses, midwives and nursing associates.* http://www.nmc.org.uk/globalassets/sitedocuments/nmc-publications/revised-new-nmc-code.pdf

Nursing and Midwifery Council (NMC). (2024). *Standards of proficiency for nursing associates.* Available online www.nmc.org.uk/globalassets/sitedocuments/standards/2024/standards-of-proficiency-for-nursing-associates.pdf

O'Connor, M. and Timmins, F. (2002). Using the Roper, Logan and Tierney model in a neonatal ICU. *Professional Nurse.*17(9):527–530. PMID: 12025013.

Office for Health Improvement & Disparities. (2023). *Premature mortality in adults with severe mental illness.*

Office for National Statistics. (2024). *Life expectancy for local areas of Great Britain: Between 2001 to 2003 and 2021 to 2023.* Available Life expectancy for local areas of Great Britain - Office for National Statistics.

Orem D.E. (2001). *Nursing: Concepts of practice,* 5th ed. St Louis: CV Mosby.

Pinto-Meza, A., Serrano-Blanco, A., Peñarrubia, M. T., Blanco, E. and Haro, J. M. (2005). Assessing depression in primary care with the PHQ-9: Can it be carried out over the telephone? *Journal of General Internal Medicine.* 20(8):738–742. https://doi.org/10.1111/j.1525-1497.2005.0144.x. PMID: 16050884; PMCID: PMC1490180.

Public Health England. (2018). *Severe mental illness (SMI) and physical health inequalities-briefing.* Available online: www.gov.uk/government/publications/severe-mental-illness-smi-physical-health-inequalities/severe-mental-illness-and-physical-health-inequalities-briefing

Public Health England. (2019). *Health matters: Health and work – guidance.* Available online: www.gov.uk/government/publications/health-matters-health-and-work/health-matters-health-and-work

Re: B. (*Adult:* Refusal of Medical Treatment). (2002). *2 All England Reports 449.* https://vlex.co.uk/vid/re-b-adult-refusal-793509269 (Accessed 15 October 2025).

Re: C. (Adult: Refusal of Treatment). (1994). *1 All ER 819.* https://www.scribd.com/document/796368494/In-re-C-ADULT-REFUSAL-OF-TREATMENT-1994-1-WLR-290 (Accessed 15 October 2025).

Resar R., Griffin F.A., Haraden C. and Nolan T. W. (2001). Using care bundles to improve health care quality. *IHI Innovation Series white paper.* Cambridge, Massachusetts: Institute for Healthcare Improvement; 2012.

Resus.org (2024). *The ABCDE approach.* Available online: www.resus.org.uk/library/abcde-approach (Accessed 26 October 2024).

Riskin, A., Erez, A., Foulk, T. A., Kugelma, A., Gover, A., Shoris, I., Riskin, K. S. and Bamberger, P. A. (2015). The impact of rudeness on medical team performance: A randomized trial. *Pediatrics,* 136(3):487–495.

Robb, Y. A. (1997). Have nursing models a place in intensive care units? *Intensive and Critical Care Nursing,* 13:93–98.

Robinson, J., Raphael, D., Moeke-Maxwell, T., Parr, J., Gott, M. and Slark, J. (2024). Implementing interventions to improve compassionate nursing care: A literature review. *International Nursing Review,* 71:457–467. https://doi.org/10.1111/inr.12910

Roper N., Logan W. and Tierney A. (2000). *The elements of nursing.* Edinburgh: Churchill Livingstone.

Rothman, M. J., Solinger, A. B., Rothman, S. I. and Finlay G. D. (2012). Clinical implications and validity of nursing assessments: A longitudinal measure of patient condition from analysis of the Electronic Medical Record. *British Medical Journal Open.* http://doi.org10.1136/bmjopen-2012-000849

Royal College of Nursing. (2023). *Career resource for registered nurses.* Available at: www.rcn.org.uk/Professional-Development/Nursing-careers-resource (Accessed 01 October 2024).

Royal College of Nursing. (2024). *New analysis reveals devastating collapse in learning disability nursing workforce.*

Royal College of Physicians. (2017). *National Early Warning Score (NEWS) 2: Standardising the assessment of acute-illness severity in the NHS. Updated report of a working party.* London: RCP.

Rush, A. J., Gullion, C. M., Basco, M. R., Jarrett, R. B. and Trivedi, M. H. (1996). The inventory of depressive symptomatology (IDS): Psychometric properties. *Psychological Medicine,* 26(3): 477–486.

Scally, G. and Donaldson, L. J. (1989). Looking forward: Clinical governance and the drive for quality improvement in the new NHS in England. *British Medical Journal,* 317:61–65.

Social Care Institute for Excellence. (2021). *Joint needs assessment and care planning – activities to achieve integrated care.* www.scie.org.uk/integrated-care/research-practice/activities/joint-needs-assessment-care-planning/

Spitzer, R. L., Kroenke, K., Williams, J. B. and Löwe, B. (2006). A brief measure for assessing generalized anxiety disorder: The GAD-7. *Archives of Internal Medicine,* 166(10):1092–1097.

Standing, M. (2008). Clinical judgement and decision-making in nursing - nine modes of practice in a revised cognitive continuum. *J Adv Nurs.*, Apr; 62(1):124–34. https://doi.org/10.1111/j.1365-2648.2007.04583.x. PMID: 18352971.

Strauss, C., Taylor, B. L., Gu, J., Baer, R., Jones, F. and Cavanagh, K. (2016). What is compassion and how can we measure it? A review of definitions and measures. *Clinical Psychology Review*, 47:15–27.

Trzeciak, S. and Mazzarelli, A. (2019). *Compassionomics: The revolutionary scientific evidence that caring makes a difference.* Pensacola, Florida: Studer Group.

Turner, A. (2017). Poor multi-agency working a factor in case where self-neglecting women died. *Community Care.* www.communitycare.co.uk/2017/11/08/poor-multi-agency-working-factor-case-self-neglecting-woman-died/

Vanhaecht, K. (2007). *The impact of clinical pathways on the organisation of care processes.*

Warren, M. A. (1973). On the moral and legal status of abortion. *The Monist*, 57(1): 43–61.

Wastell, C. and Howarth, S. (2022). *Reasoning, judging, deciding: The science of thinking.* United Kingdom: SAGE Publications Ltd.

Waterlow, J. (1985). Pressure sores: A risk assessment card. *Nursing Times.* 81(48):49–55. PMID: 3853163.

West, M. A. and Dawson, J. F. (2012). *Employee engagement and NHS performance.* [online] Available at: www.kingsfund.org.uk/sites/default/files/employee-engagement-nhs-performance-west-dawson-leadership-review2012-paper.pdf

West, M., Bailey, S. and Williams, E. (2020). *The courage of compassion supporting nurses and midwives to deliver high-quality care.* London: Kings Fund.

West, M. A. (2021). *Compassionate leadership: Sustaining wisdom, humanity and presence in health and social care.* Swirling Leaf Press.

WHO. (2024). *Improving early childhood development.* Geneva: WHO Guideline World Health Organization.

Williams, B (2022). The national early warning score: From concept to NHS Implementation. *Clinical Medicine*, 22(6): 499–505.

Wong, D. and Baker, C. (1998). Pain in children: Comparison of assessment scales. *Pediatric Nursing*, 14(1):9–17.

World Health Organization (WHO). (1946). *Constitution of the World Health Organisation.* WHO: Geneva.

World Health Organization (WHO). (2007). *Communication during patient hand-overs.* Switzerland. WHO Press. Available online: https://cdn.who.int/media/docs/default-source/patient-safety/patient-safety-solutions/ps-solution3-communication-during-patient-handovers.pdf?sfvrsn=7a54c664_8

World Health Organization (WHO). (2018). *WHO housing and health guidelines.* World Health Organization, Geneva. Available at: https://www.who.int/publications/i/item/9789241550376

World Health Organization (WHO). (2022). *How can skill-mix innovations support the implementation of integrated care for people with chronic conditions and multimorbidity? Policy Brief 46.* Copenhagen: WHO.

World Health Organization (WHO). (2023). *Improving early childhood development.* Geneva: WHO Guideline World Health Organization.

World Health Organization (WHO) (2024). *Constitution.* Available online at: www.who.int/about/accountability/governance/constitution (last accessed 7 May 2024).

Young, M., Thomas, A., Lubarsky, S., Ballard, T., Gordon, D., Gruppen, L. D., Holmboe, E., Ratcliffe, T., Rencic, J., Schuwirth, L. and Durning, S. J. (2018). Drawing boundaries: The difficulty in defining clinical reasoning. *Academic Medicine*, 93(7): 990–995. https://doi.org/10.1097/ACM. 0000000000002142

Yura, H. and Walsh, M. (1967). *The nursing process.* Norwalk: Appleton- Century- Crofts.

Index

A

Abortion, 11

Accountability, 1–2, 6

    accountable practice links to assessing, planning and monitoring care, 18–21

    act professionally and importance of evidence-based thinking, 15–16

    back to personhood quickly, 13

    best interests concept, 9–10

    interesting legal cases help determine impact of personhood in healthcare, 12

    means to be answerable, 7–9

    Penny case study, 5

    person-centred and holistic care, 13–15

    personhood concept, 11–13

    policies and ethical frameworks, 16–17

    regulatory and governance requirements, 16–17

    responsibility and delegation and links to assessment and planning, 6–7

    understand and apply relevant legal, 16–17

Accountable practice links to assessing, planning and monitoring care, 18–21

Activities of daily living (ADLs), 90, 95

Act professionally and importance of evidence-based thinking, 15–16

Adoo-Kissi-Debrah, E., 120–121

Adult, 24

    nursing disciplines, 49–50

Adulthood, 50, 114

Advance decision, 135–137

Advance statement, 136–137

Adverse Childhood Experiences (ACEs), 50

Age, 46

Ahmed, Z., 129–130

Airedale National Health Service Trust v Bland (1993), 12

Airway, Breathing, Circulation, Disability, Exposure approach (ABCDE approach), 79–80, 85

Aldridge, J., 98–99

Alert, 86

Analytical thinking, 77–78

Anxiety disorders, 67

Artificial nutrition, 12

Aseptic non-touch technique (ANTT), 78

ASPIRE, 91, 93

Assessing care, accountable practice links to, 18–21

Assessment, 6, 15, 33–34, 62–63, 91, 99

accountability, responsibility and delegation and links to, 6–7

    findings, 6

    informs care plans, 1

Assessment, planning, implementation and evaluation (APIE), 90–91, 98–99

Assessment tools, 58, 63, 68–69, 74, 85

    Adrianna case study, 57

    benefits and limitations of, 69–72

    importance of using assessment tools in practice, 63–69

    Meena case study, 57

    purpose of, 58–61

    registered nursing associate voice, 57

    risk assessment tools, 61–62

    screening tools or screening instruments, 58–61

    sensitivity and specificity of tests, 59

    understanding, 2

    understanding terms associated with, 62–63

Attorney, lasting power of, 137–138

Autonomy, 17

B

'Baby P', 31

Bailey, S., 130

Battey, B., 54

Beauchamp, T. L., 17, 33

Beneficence, 17

Benner, P., 80

Best interests, concept of, 9–10

Biological, psychological and social model (BPS model), 41

Biomedical ethics, 17

Biopsychosocial (BPS)

    model, 40, 45, 53–54, 58, 110

    needs, 98–99

    nursing associate role in providing BPS care, 48–49

    protected characteristics and, 45–46

Bio-psycho-social healthcare assessment, 2

    bio-psycho-social model and person-centred care, 45

    historical overview, 40–44

    housing, 42–44

    protected characteristics and bio-psycho-social model, 45–46

    role of nursing associate in providing bio-psycho-social care, 48–49

separate disciplines, 49–53
social prescribing, 46–48
spiritual model, 53–55
Body mass index (BMI), 57
Breast screening, 58–59
Brief Pain Inventory (BPI), 65–66
Brief Pain Inventory shortened form (BPI-sf), 65–66
Burn-out, 127, 130

C
Cardiopulmonary resuscitation (CPR), 135
Cardiovascular disease, 50–51
Care, 30
    importance of care coordination, 28–32
    plans, 18–21
Care bundles, 62, 101, 103, 108
    challenges to, 103
    sepsis six care bundle, 90
Care pathways, 101, 103–104, 108
    advantages of, 104–108
Care Quality Commission (CQC), 16
Caring society, 118
Central venous access devices (CVC), 102
Challenge, 86
Cheetham, L. J. E., 133
Child, 24, 49–50
Childhood trauma, 50
Children, 50, 114
Childress, J. F., 17, 33
Chiumento, A., 130
Chronic Pulmonary Obstructive Disease (COPD),
    50–51
Civility, 33–34
Civil partnership, 46
Climbié, V., 31
Clinical algorithms, 62
Clinical decision-making, 69, 72, 76, 81
Clinical governance, 17
Clinical judgement, 69–72
Clinical reasoning, 76, 79, 81
    five rights of, 76
    Jay case study, 73
Clinical settings, 67
Clinical skills, 82–83
Cognitive continuum theory, 79–80
Commercial activity, 113
Common morality, 17
Communication, 26, 52–53, 82–83, 87
Community
    community-based MDTs, 29
    learning disability, 99
    nursing team, 115
    services, 117–118
Compassion, 33–34, 126, 128, 131–132
    advance decision, 135–137
    compassion-fatigue, 130
    especially important, 134–138
    lasting power of attorney, 137–138
    matter, 128–130
    matter #2, 138–139
    Peter case study, 125

Compassionate assessment importance for people, 3
Compassionate care, 126
    compassionate cultures ensure, 132–133
Compassionate cultures, 3
    ensure compassionate care, 132–133
Compassionate nursing care, 129–130
Compassionate principles, assessing and planning
    based on, 130–132
Competency, 80
Connelly, P., 31
Conversations, 10
'Core20', 118–119
Core20PLUS5 programme, 118–120
COVID-19 pandemic, 31, 121, 130
Crimean war, 93

D
Dahlgren, G., 3, 113
Dahlgren-Whitehead model, 112
Data, 69
Decision-making, 79, 85
    Jay case study, 73
    system one and system two thinking, 75–76
    understanding, 74–76
Deep-vein thrombosis (DVT), 27
Delegation to assessment and planning, 6–7
Department of Health and Social Care, 115
Depression severity scores, 67–68
Depressive symptoms, 67
Descriptive decision-making, 73
Descriptive theory, 77
Disability, 46
Donaldson, L. J., 17
Dreyfus, S. E., 80
'Duty of care', 8

E
Economic environment, 113
Edinburgh Postnatal Depression Scale (EPDS), 66
Educational resources, 46
Effective care, 27
Effective health screening, 58–59
Electrocardiogram (ECG), 84
Emergency, 86
Emotional intelligence, 82
Employing organisation, 8
Empowering patients, 130–131
Equality Act (2010), 45–46
Escalate care, 2, 86
    RSVP, 85–88
    SBARD approach, 85
    tools for monitoring and escalating patient care,
        85–88
    understanding clinical reasoning and clinical
        decision-making, 76–81
    understanding decision-making, 74–76
Escalating patient care, tools for, 85–88
Ethical frameworks, 17
Ethnic minority communities, 119
Euthanasia, 11

Evaluation, 91
Evidence-based interventions, 101
Evidence-based thinking, act professionally and importance of, 15–16
Excellent care, 12
Expert, novice to, 80–81
External factors, 74

F
'Faces' pain rating scale, 64
Faith, 46
Falls risk assessment tool (FRAT), 62
False negatives, 59
False positives, 59
Family-centred care, 100
    personhood leads to, 24–26
'Five rights' of clinical reasoning, 76

G
Gender
    identity, 11
    reassignment, 46
Generalised Anxiety Disorder 7 (GAD-7), 63, 67
Getting it right first time (GIRFT), 90, 103
Gibbs, G., 98–99
    model of reflection, 69
Gilbert, P., 126
Glasper, A., 16
Good teamwork, 81, 83
Griffiths model, 90, 98, 101
    Aubrey case study, 89

H
Hammond, K. R., 79
Harris, M., 13
Health, 41, 81, 110, 137–138
    deprivation, 28
    Jenny case study, 109
    main determinants of, 112–113
    service planners, 111
    wider determinants of, 3, 110, 113
    wider/social determinants impact on health outcomes for individuals and communities, 114–118
Health and Care Act, 32
Healthcare, 8
    interesting legal cases help determine impact of personhood in, 12
    professionals, 28, 45, 49, 54, 77, 101, 110, 126, 130
    services, 130–131
    staff, 8
Health Education England, 29
Health equality framework (HEF), 98–99
Health Foundation, 14, 26–27, 116–117
Health inequalities, 28, 110–111, 120–121
    managed at national and local level, 118–120
    not just urban problem, 120–121
    wider costs of, 118–121
Health screening, 58–60

in United Kingdom, 59
Henderson, V., 93–94
Heuristics, 75–76
High populations, 120–121
Hobson, S., 31
Holistic care, 13, 15, 53–54, 126
Hope, Organised Religion, Personal spiritual practice, Effects on your Care (HOPE), 54
Housing, 42–44
    differences between urban and rural areas, 42
    Joan case study, 39
    stock, 120
'Human', 11
    existence, 74
    needs model, 90, 95, 97
    Sam case study, 89
Humanistic approach, 41
Hydration, 12
Hypertension, 120

I
Ill-health, 114
Implementation, 91, 99
Incivility, 133
'Inclusion health groups', 111–112
Inclusivity, 33–34
Index of Multiple Deprivation (IMD), 118–119
Individual care, 1
Individual healthcare professionals, 30
Information, 110–111
Insomnia, 92
Integrated care
    meant by, 32–33
    systems, 32
Integrated care boards (ICBs), 117–118
Integrated working, 30–31
Interagency care, 30, 32
    Shahida case study, 23
Internal factors, 74
Interprofessional care, 29–30, 32
Interprofessional liaison and care, 30
Interprofessional working, 29–30
Inter-rater reliability, 62–63
Intra-reliability, 62–63
Intuition originates, 79
Intuition thinking, 77–78
Irritable Bowel Syndrome, 50–51

J
Judgement process, 76
Justice, 17

K
Kahneman, D., 75, 80

L
Landmark decision, 120–121
Language matters, 6

Index

Lasting Power of Attorney (LPA), 137
Leaders, 129–130
Learning, 24
    features, 3–4
Learning disability (LD), 28, 49–51, 53, 98–99
    Ben case study, 39
    mortality review, 28
Life-sustaining treatment, 135
Links to assessment and planning, 6–7
Living will, 135
Logan W., 95

M
Malenfant, S., 127
Marriage, 46
Maternity, 46
McCance, T., 98–99
McCormack, B., 98–99
McGill Pain Questionnaire (MPQ), 65
Mead, M., 129
Mental Capacity Act, The (MCA), 5, 9, 135
Mental health, 24, 49–51
    condition, 114
    services, 31
Mental illness, 12
Mental short cuts, 75–76
Mental State Examination (MSE), 68–69
Midwives, 6
Mild learning disability, 25
Mini-mental state examination (MMSE), 68–69
Monitor care, 2
    accountable practice links to, 18–21
    RSVP, 85–88
    SBARD approach, 85
    tools for monitoring and escalating patient care,
        85–88
    tools for monitoring patient care, 85–88
    understanding clinical reasoning and clinical
        decision-making, 76–81
    understanding decision-making, 74–76
Motor Neurone Disease (MND), 136
Moulster model, 90, 98, 101
    Aubrey case study, 89
Multi-agency
    approach, 31
    working, 31
Multidimensional assessment scales, 64–65
Multidimensional pain assessment scales, 65
Multi-disciplinary care, 32
Multi-disciplinary team (MDT), 1–2, 24, 29–30

N
National Early Warning Score 2 (NEWS2), 62
National Health Service (NHS), 40, 58–59
    Long Term Plan, 45
National Healthcare Inequalities Improvement
    Programme, 28
National Institute for Health and Care Excellence
    (NICE), 16, 61, 101, 138
National screening programmes, 58–59

Nightingale, F., 93
Non-invasive ventilation (NIV), 136
Non-maleficence, 17
Normative decision-making, 73
Numerical pain assessment scales, 64–65
Numerical pain rating scale (NPRS), 62, 64
Numerical rating scale (NRS), 64
Numerical scale, 64
Nurses, 6, 8, 17, 51
    intuition, 79
Nursing, 6, 24
    care, 18, 21, 47, 94
    diagnosis, 92
    practice, 80
    system, 97–98
    workforce cares, 130–131
Nursing and Midwifery Council (NMC), 1, 3, 6
    requirements for NMC standards of proficiency for
        NAs, 3
Nursing associates (NAs), 1–2, 6, 45, 47, 49–50, 52,
        84, 126
    requirements for NMC standards of proficiency
        for, 3
    role in providing bio-psycho-social care, 48–49
Nursing Associate Curriculum Framework, 110
Nursing models, 90, 93–94
    human needs model, 95–97
    Moulster and Griffiths model, 98–101
    self-care model, 97–98
    understanding, 93–101
Nursing process, 90–91, 93
    APIE, 91
    ASPIRE, 91
    principles of, 90–93
    Ronnie case study, 89

O
Office for Health Improvements and Disparities
    (OHID), 115, 121
Office for National Statistics (ONS), 116–117
Orem D. E., 98–99
    self-care model, 91, 97
Organisations, 103

P
Parkinson's disease, 30
Partnership, working in, 26
    with people, 2
Patient Healthcare Questionnaire (PHQ-9), 67–68
Patients, 17, 47, 54, 133
People
    Brenda case study, 23
    sensitive and compassionate assessment and
        planning importance for, 3
    things to, 26–28
Percutaneous endoscopic gastrostomy (PEG), 136
Peripheral access devices (PVC), 102
'Person', 10–11
    care, 28–29
Personal experiences, 10

Person-centred care, 13, 15, 45
  Eshan case study, 5
  four principles of, 6–7
  personhood leads to, 24–26
Personhood, 10, 14
  back to personhood quickly, 13
  concept of, 11–13
  Harry case study, 23
  interesting legal cases help determine impact of
      personhood in healthcare, 12
  leads to person-and family-centred care, 24–26
Planning, 6, 91
  accountability, responsibility and delegation and
      links to, 6–7
  accountable practice links to planning care 18–21
  importance for people, 3
  individualised care, 126
Planning nursing care
  care bundles and care pathways, 101–108
  principles and theories of, 2
  principles of nursing process, 90–93
  understanding nursing models, 93–101
'PLUS', 119
Poor mental health, 117
Post-traumatic stress disorder, 67
Pregnancy, 46
Prescriptive decision-making, 73
Pressure Ulcer Risk Primary or Secondary Evaluation
    Tool (PURPOSE-T), 61
Primary care, 29
Probe, 86
Probe, alert, challenge, escalate (PACE), 86
Problem-solving process, 90
Professional body, 7
Professional practice, 16
Proficiency, 80
  requirements for NMC standards of proficiency for
      NAs, 3
Psychological factors, 40
Public Health England (PHE), 117, 121
Public Health Observatory, 100

R
Race, 46
Radioactive dye, 60
Rainbow model, 113
Reason, Story, Vital Signs, Plan (RSVP), 85–85
  Sam case study, 73
Recheck, 91–93
Recipient experiences, 133
'Red tape', 32
Reflection, 99
Reflective activity, 10
Refuse treatment, 135
Registered nurses (RNs), 6
  different levels of responsibility for, 90
  key differences between and RNA and, 6–7
Registered Nursing Associate (RNA), 2, 6, 18, 21, 24,
    58, 60, 68–69, 72, 74–75, 90, 117
  different levels of responsibility for, 90
  key differences between and RN and, 6–7

Relevant proficiencies, 3
Reliability, 62
Religion, 46
Responsibility to assessment and planning, 6–7
Right action, 78, 84
Right cues, 77–78, 84
Right patient, 78, 84
Right reason, 78, 84
Right time, 78, 84
Risk assessment tools, 57, 61–62
  clinical algorithms, 62
Riskin, A., 133
Robinson, J., 129–130
Roper N., 95
Royal College of Nursing (RCN), 17, 24, 51

S
SARS-CoV-2
  pandemic, 67–68
  pathogen, 116
Scally, G., 17
Screening instruments, 58–61
  Aadhya case study, 57
Screening programmes, 60
Screening tools, 58–61
  Aadhya case study, 57
Second World War, 40
Secondary care, 29
Self-care, 98
  deficit, 98
Self-care model, 97–98
  of nursing, 90
  Remy case study, 89
Sensitive assessment importance for people, 3
Separate disciplines, 49–53
  child, 50
  LD, 51–53
  mental health, 50–51
Sex, 46
Sexual orientation, 46
Shortened Form-McGill Pain Questionnaire
    (SF-MPQ), 65
'Silo' working, 29
Situation, background, assessment, recommendation,
    decision approach (SBARD approach), 85
Social anxiety disorder, 67
Social care, 81
Social Care Institute for Excellence, 29
Social-cultural environment, 50
Social determinants, 110
  impact on health outcomes for individuals and
      communities, 114–118
Social environment, 113
Social factors, 40
Social prescribing, 46, 48, 117–118
  factors that impact person's quality of life, 41
  Joan case study, 39
Social security system, 40
Socioeconomic factors, 110
'Soft skill', 126, 129–130
Spiritual care, 54

Index

Spirituality, 53–54
Spiritual model, 53–55
Spiritual nursing care theory model, 54
Staff focus, 17
Standards of Proficiency for Nursing Associates, 14–15
Steele, A., 31
Stephens, B., 27
Stress, sustained levels of, 50
Stroke, 50–51
Student Nursing Associates (SNAs), 1–2, 6, 18, 21, 24, 49–50, 58, 60, 68–69, 72, 75, 90, 117
Substantial employment, 114
Systematic nursing diagnosis, 91

T
Teamwork, 81–82
Textbooks, 3–4
Thumb, rules of, 75–76
Tierney A., 95
Tracer, 60
'Track and trigger' systems, 2
Transformational leadership, 129–130
Turner, C., 133

U
UK National Screening Committee (UK NSC), 58–59
Underpinning theory, 90
Unemployment
    impact of, 114
    in adulthood, 114
United Kingdom, 101, 121
Urban decay, 120

V
Validity, 62
Verbal pain assessment scales, 64–65

Verbal rating scale (VRS), 64–65
Vicarious liability, 8–9
Visual analogue scale (VAS), 64
Visual pain assessment scales, 64–65

W
Walsh, M., 90–91
Warren, M. A., 11
Welfare, 137–138
Welfare State, 40
West, M., 130
Whitehead, M., 3, 113
Wider determinants, 110
    Avery case study, 109
    of health, 110–113
    impact on health outcomes for individuals and communities, 114–118
    Jenny case study, 109
    Luca case study, 109
    model to help understand, 112–113
Wider multi-disciplinary team, understanding your role in, 81–84
    Jay case study, 73
    registered nurse associate voice, 73
    working collaboratively, 73
Williams, B., 16
Williams, E., 130
Work experiences, 10
Working
    benefits of, 83–84
    in partnership, 2, 26, 45
World Health Organization (WHO), 15–16, 29, 41, 50, 85, 101

Y
Yura, H., 90–91